The Washington
Manual™ Surgery
Survival Guide

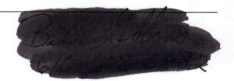

The Washington Manual™ Surgery Survival Guide

Faculty Advisors

Bruce Lee Hall, M.D., Ph.D., M.B.A.
Assistant Professor of Surgery
Adjunct Professor of Business Administration
Washington University School of Medicine
Barnes-Jewish Hospital
St. Louis, Missouri

Sanjeev Bhalla, M.D.
Assistant Professor of Radiology
Mallinckrodt Institute of Radiology
Barnes-Jewish Hospital
St. Louis, Missouri

Mark S. Weinfeld, M.D.
Assistant Professor of Medicine
Department of Internal Medicine
Cardiovascular Division
Washington University School of Medicine
Barnes-Jewish Hospital
St. Louis, Missouri

The Washington Manual™ Surgery Survival Guide

Editors

Jeremy Goodman, M.D.
Resident in General Surgery
Department of Surgery
Washington University School of Medicine
Barnes-Jewish Hospital
St. Louis, Missouri

Nirmal K. Veeramachaneni, M.D.
Resident in Surgery
Department of Surgery
Washington University School of Medicine
Barnes-Jewish Hospital
St. Louis, Missouri

Emily R. Winslow, M.D.
Resident in General Surgery
Department of Surgery
Washington University School of Medicine
Barnes-Jewish Hospital
St. Louis, Missouri

Series Editor

Tammy L. Lin, M.D.
Adjunct Assistant Professor of Medicine
Washington University School of Medicine
St. Louis, Missouri

Series Advisor

Daniel M. Goodenberger, M.D.
Professor of Medicine
Chief, Division of Medical Education
Washington University School of Medicine
Director, Internal Medicine Residency Program
Barnes-Jewish Hospital
St. Louis, Missouri

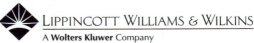
LIPPINCOTT WILLIAMS & WILKINS
A **Wolters Kluwer** Company
Philadelphia · Baltimore · New York · London
Buenos Aires · Hong Kong · Sydney · Tokyo

Acquisitions Editors: Danette Knopp and James Ryan
Developmental Editors: Scott Marinaro and Keith Donnellan
Supervising Editor: Mary Ann McLaughlin
Production Editor: Erica Broennle Nelson, Silverchair Science + Communications
Manufacturing Manager: Colin Warnock
Cover Designer: QT Design
Compositor: Silverchair Science + Communications
Printer: Victor Graphics

©2003 by Department of Medicine, Washington University School of Medicine

Library of Congress Cataloging-in-Publication Data
Goodman, Jeremy.
   The Washington manual surgery survival guide / Jeremy Goodman, Nirmal K. Veeramachaneni, Emily R. Winslow.
      p. ; cm. -- (Washington manual survival guide series)
   Includes index.
   ISBN 0-7817-4368-0
   1. Surgery--Handbooks, manuals, etc. 2. Surgery--Study and teaching
(Residency)--Handbooks, manuals, etc. 3. Residency (Medicine)--Handbooks, manuals,
etc. I. Veeramachaneni, Nirmal K. II. Winslow, Emily R. III. Title. IV. Series.
   [DNLM: 1. Surgical Procedures, Minor--methods--Handbooks. 2. Internship and
Residency--Handbooks. WO 39 G653w 2003]
RD37.G665 2003
617--dc21

2003044666

The Washington Manual™ is an intent-to-use mark belonging to Washington University in St. Louis to which international legal protection applies. The mark is used in this publication by LWW under license from Washington University.
   Care has been taken to confirm the accuracy of the information presented and to describe generally accepted practices. However, the authors, editors, and publisher are not responsible for errors or omissions or for any consequences from application of the information in this book and make no warranty, expressed or implied, with respect to the currency, completeness, or accuracy of the contents of the publication. Application of this information in a particular situation remains the professional responsibility of the practitioner.
   The authors, editors, and publisher have exerted every effort to ensure that drug selection and dosage set forth in this text are in accordance with current recommendations and practice at the time of publication. However, in view of ongoing research, changes in government regulations, and the constant flow of information relating to drug therapy and drug reactions, the reader is urged to check the package insert for each drug for any change in indications and dosage and for added warnings and precautions. This is particularly important when the recommended agent is a new or infrequently employed drug.
   Some drugs and medical devices presented in this publication have Food and Drug Administration (FDA) clearance for limited use in restricted research settings. It is the responsibility of health care providers to ascertain the FDA status of each drug or device planned for use in their clinical practice.

10 9 8 7 6 5 4 3 2 1

Contents

CONTENTS

VI. COMMON PROBLEMS

VII. CRITICAL CARE

CONTENTS

Contributing Authors

Sam B. Bhayani, M.D.
Instructor of Urology
Brady Urological Institute
Johns Hopkins University School
  of Medicine
Baltimore, Maryland

Raja Dhalla, M.D.
Resident in Orthopaedic Surgery
Department of Orthopaedic Surgery
Washington University School
  of Medicine
Barnes-Jewish Hospital
St. Louis, Missouri

Douglas John Fox, Jr., M.D.
Resident in Neurosurgery
Department of Neurosurgery
Washington University School
  of Medicine
St. Louis, Missouri

Jeremy Goodman, M.D.
Resident in General Surgery
Department of Surgery
Washington University School
  of Medicine
Barnes-Jewish Hospital
St. Louis, Missouri

Aaron G. Grand, M.D.
Resident
Department of Surgery
Division of Plastic and Recon-
  structive Surgery
Washington University School
  of Medicine
St. Louis, Missouri

Ravi Gurujal, M.D.
Fellow in Cardiology
Department of Cardiology
Washington University School
  of Medicine
St. Louis, Missouri

Eric C. Leuthardt, M.D.
Senior Resident
Department of Neurological Surgery
Washington University School of
  Medicine
Barnes-Jewish Hospital
St. Louis, Missouri

Joseph V. Philip, M.D.
Clinical Assistant
Department of Radiology
Massachusetts General Hospital
Boston, Massachusetts

Nirmal K. Veeramachaneni, M.D.
Resident in Surgery
Department of Surgery
Washington University School
  of Medicine
Barnes-Jewish Hospital
St. Louis, Missouri

Benjamin W. Verdine, M.D.
Resident
Department of Surgery
Division of Plastic and Recon-
  structive Surgery
Washington University School
  of Medicine
Barnes-Jewish Hospital
St. Louis, Missouri

Emily R. Winslow, M.D.
Resident in General Surgery
Department of Surgery
Washington University School
  of Medicine
Barnes-Jewish Hospital
St. Louis, Missouri

Chairman's Note

Medical knowledge is increasing at an exponential rate, and physicians are being bombarded with new facts at a pace that many find overwhelming. The Washington Manual™ Survival Guides were developed in this context for interns, residents, medical students, and other practitioners in need of readily accessible practical clinical information. They therefore meet an important need in an era of information overload.

I would like to acknowledge the authors who have contributed to these books. In particular, Tammy L. Lin, M.D., Series Editor, provided energetic and inspired leadership, and Daniel M. Goodenberger, M.D., Series Advisor, Chief of the Division of Medical Education in the Department of Medicine at Washington University, is a continual source of sage advice. The efforts and outstanding skill of the lead authors are evident in the quality of the final product. I am confident that this series will meet its desired goal of providing practical knowledge that can be directly applied to improving patient care.

Kenneth S. Polonsky, M.D.
Adolphus Busch Professor
Chairman, Department of Medicine
Washington University School of Medicine
St. Louis, Missouri

Series Preface

The Washington Manual™ Survival Guides, a multispecialty series, is designed to provide interns, residents, medical students, or anyone on the front lines of clinical care with quick, practical, essential information in an accessible format. It lets you hit the ground running as you learn the basics of practicing clinical medicine, gain more responsibility, and become a valued team member. Although written individually, they all incorporate series features. Each book takes care to give you an insider's view of how to get things done efficiently and effectively, tips on how to "survive" training, and pearls you will want to pass on in the future. It is similar to receiving a great sign-out from your favorite resident. When faced with an unfamiliar situation, we envision getting timely information and guidance from the survival guide (like you would from your resident) to make appropriate decisions at 3:00 p.m. or 3:00 a.m.

One of the most unique and notable features of this new series is that it was truly a joint effort across subspecialties at Washington University. We were fortunate to have significant departmental support, particularly from Kenneth Polonsky, M.D., whose commitment made this series possible. Every survival guide has the credibility of being written by recent interns, residents, or chief residents in that specialty with input from faculty advisors. We were fortunate to have found outstanding lead authors who were not only highly regarded clinicians and teachers, but who also provided significant leadership and collaborated well together. Their incredible enthusiasm and desire to pass on their hard-earned knowledge, experiences, and wisdom clearly shine through in the series.

Anyone who has been through training will tell you the hours are long, the work is hard, and your energy is limited. With either a print or electronic version of a survival guide by your side, we hope you will work more efficiently, make decisions with more confidence, stay out of trouble, and get that ever-elusive good night's rest.

Tammy L. Lin, M.D., Series Editor
Daniel M. Goodenberger, M.D., Series Advisor

Preface

A surgical internship promises to be one of the most trying experiences of your life. Yet with all of the nonstop days and sleepless nights comes the immense satisfaction of a job well done. You are finally responsible for another person's well-being: It's a daunting prospect to say the least, but, rest assured, you have the skills and the knowledge to succeed.

At times you may feel alone; that's why we've written this book for you. Your chief resident will tell you to discharge a patient but probably won't take the time to explain *how*. The nurse who calls you at 2:00 a.m. expects an answer, not a puzzled expression. The attending expects the preops to be ready for the day's surgeries. At the end of your internship year, these scenarios will seem like child's play. But everyone needs a little help in the beginning.

Turn to this book to help you through your daily grind. Cross out those details that don't apply at your institution. Make notes in the margins. Keep it close at hand: It represents the collective knowledge of interns who have come before you.

We also welcome medical students, whether fresh from Step 1 or starting an advanced surgery clerkship. The more you can act like an intern, the smoother things will go for the patients and the team, and the greater the benefits you'll derive from your rotation. This book can propel you out of the ranks of the average medical student and into the realm of the junior house officer.

As difficult as it can be, surgery provides a healthy dose of fun. Concentrate on the positive aspects of what you are doing. Routine cases will at times become complex, and patients with even the simplest of diseases can harbor fascinating pathology. If you don't look carefully, you may miss the forest for the trees. Keep your eyes and your mind open, and you're in for the time of your life.

We would like to thank the many people involved in the review of this book: Suzanne Albrecht, Jerry Chang, Li Erin Chen, Jeffrey Drebin, Ashley Flynn, Paul Frohnert, Courtney Gelberman, Pat Geraghty, Jennifer Heaton, David Kawamura, Mary Klingensmith, Kelly Koay, Amy Lawson, Heather Mahoney, Yosuke Miyahshita, Valerie Montalvo, Brent Ragar, Anne Renfro, Susan Rider, Jared Smith, Cylburn Soden, Tim Stark, LeRoi Stephenson, Toms Sviskrski, Casey Swenson, Michele Tang, Eric Volckmann, and Katherine Yung. The editors extend special thanks to faculty advisors Bruce Hall, Sanjeev Bhalla, and Mark Weinfeld.

J.G.
N.K.V.
E.R.W.

Key to Abbreviations

AAO	awake, alert, and oriented
C & F	clear and fluent (speech)
DIP	distal interphalangeal
EOMI	extraocular muscles intact
FC	follows commands
IVP	intravenous pyelogram
KUB	kidneys, ureters, bladder
LT	light touch
MCP	metacarpophalangeal
MS	musculoskeletal
Nl	normal
PCP	phencyclidine
PERL	pupils equal and react to light
PIP	proximal interphalangeal
PSA	prostate-specific antigen
TML	tongue midline
TPN	total parenteral nutrition

1

Keys to Survival

Jeremy Goodman,
Nirmal K. Veeramachaneni,
and Emily R. Winslow

1. Never lie: Instead of making up the facts, admit you don't know the answer, and then go find it.
2. Keep a "to do" list throughout the day, and cross or check off each task once you've completed it.
3. Keep something in your pocket at all times to read during moments of downtime.
4. If you don't feel comfortable with a procedure, ask for help. Never put your own pride in the way of patient safety.
5. When you go home at night, forget about the hospital and do something you enjoy. Eat, sleep, and exercise when you can.
6. Make time for family; as difficult as your residency is, it's even harder on them.
7. Keep a change of clothes and some toiletries in your locker at the hospital.
8. Be understanding and gracious when answering consult requests. The key to a successful career is a healthy relationship with your nonsurgery colleagues.
9. Nurses are a great resource—befriend them, respect them, and learn from them.
10. Remember that your life as a surgeon is not the same as your life as a resident. You have great things to look forward to.

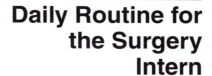

Daily Routine for the Surgery Intern

Your daily routine as an intern will vary tremendously based on the type of hospital, surgical service, and team you are working with. There are some common denominators in the day of a surgical house officer, and we address them here. The big picture is that there is always a lot to do and not enough time in which to do it. Your job is to figure out a system that allows you to manage your time so the most important problems are taken care of first, and the other problems are attended to in priority order. If you stay organized and positive, you will be amazed at how much more you can get done.

2 Organizing Your Day

Emily R. Winslow

. . . back to the daily grind . . .

SIGN OUT

In most programs, a coverage system dictates that another intern watches over your patients when you are not on call. Good communication between the regular team and the night coverage is essential.

- Meet the covering intern in the morning to exchange information. Ask if any new orders were written so you can follow up.

- If something significant happened to one of your patients overnight, check in on that patient.

- Talking with the night nurse is the best way to obtain information about what happened overnight.

PRE-ROUNDING

The term *pre-rounding* refers to preparation for morning rounds with the whole team. Pre-rounding varies from service to service, so ask your senior resident what the expectations are. At a minimum, your job will involve generating a list of patients on your service and the relevant information about them.

- For any new patients admitted overnight, review the history, physical exam, lab results, and admitting orders. Meet the patients and see if the exam and complaints have changed since admission. Doing so takes extra time but will ultimately improve your efficiency.

- Making the list is central to being an organized, efficient intern. You need to have, at a minimum, the room number, patient name, operation, postoperative day, and attending's name.

- A more complete list also includes the vital signs from the last 24 hrs. In addition, the "ins and outs" are critical in the surgical patient. "Ins" include IV fluid, PO intake, tube feeding, and TPN. "Outs" include urine output, NG output, drain output, and ostomy output.

- Know the types of tubes your patients have and how long they have been there. Also know the types of diet you have them on so you will remember to advance the diet when appropriate. Record the data in a consistent and organized fashion.

- The list can also include the current medications. It is also helpful to track the number of days the patient has been on a particular antibiotic.

- If lab results are available at the time of your pre-rounds, record them. If lab studies have been ordered but results are not available, include a notation that these will be forthcoming.

ROUNDS

The objective of rounds is to formulate a plan for each patient on your team. Your job as the intern is to make sure that the plan is executed during the day, while the rest of the team is in the OR. It is essential that you understand what the problems are and what needs to be done about them.

- During rounds, generate a complete, readable list of the things that need to be done that day. One way to make sure everything is accomplished is to leave space on the list so that you can jot things down. Draw an empty box next to each task that must be done, and fill in the box later, when the task has been completed. Remember: It is your job to make sure that the game plan is carried out correctly.

- The goal of the senior resident on rounds is to see and evaluate every patient and decide if anyone is developing a complication. To do so, the senior resident must examine every patient. Often, this means changing the dressing at the bedside. Make sure supplies are readily available to redress the wound. Using a portable "dressing cart" is helpful.

- Chart use during rounds is helpful so you can write orders and sometimes even notes during the course of rounding. This will save you time and get important orders implemented sooner than if you wait until after rounds to do all the writing.

NOTES

The chart is a legal record and should be treated as such. It should clearly convey what is happening with your patient.

- Your notes should always include a plan for the day and indicate the reason for any deviation from the routine. For example, if your patient is getting a CT scan to rule out abscess because of fever and slow return of bowel function, include this information in your note.

- Patients may also have a medical doctor following them in the hospital; you can use the chart to communicate with them. Thus, your writing must be legible.

- When you write, your notes will vary. It is best to write your notes before or during rounds so you may start taking care of new orders as soon as rounds are over.

CALLING CONSULTS

Although surgeons pride themselves on being able to care for all manner of patients, there are times when expert assistance is needed. We call on consultants to answer specific questions, assist in management, and sometimes assume primary responsibility for a patient's care. If calling a consult is your idea, make sure to check with your senior resident or attending for approval. *Also, before calling a consult, let the patient know that you have asked another physician to see him or her.*

When to Call

As an intern or junior resident, you are usually asked to call a consult by your senior resident or attending. Don't be afraid, however, to suggest consulting a specialist if you think it is in the patient's best interest.

- For patients with comorbidities, engaging the help of a specialist who treats that specific disease can be very helpful.

- Patients with rare or unusual conditions will benefit from a consultant's involvement.

- *Place your consult request as early in the day as possible*; this gives your consultant more time to see the patient and respond. Remember, however, that the consultant will not appreciate a call at 6:45 a.m. Most medical services do not switch to the daytime team until about 8:00 a.m. Bear in mind that some consultants do not work on weekends, and late Friday consults may be deferred until Monday.

- Avoid "curbsiding," the practice of informally asking suggestions of consultants. Ask for a formal consultation, which ensures proper documentation and follow-through and is medicolegally necessary.

Whom to Call

If a patient is already under the care of a specialist for a particular problem, that physician should be contacted first to help deal with the problem. Otherwise, most teaching hospitals have consult services for each specialty, and a central number or the paging operator can connect you to the appropriate person. Hospitals without formal consult services often have a list of on-call physicians from each specialty.

What Information to Have Available

When calling, be sure to provide the patient's name, date of birth, and room number; your name and pager number; the attending's name; and specific reason for consultation. Some consultants or answering services will ask your opinion on the timing of a response. Does this patient need to be seen emergently? Can he or she be seen later in the day or even tomorrow? Be familiar with the patient's general medical history, reason for hospitalization, and any procedures that have been performed.

Also, know specifics that pertain to the condition necessitating the consult. For example, you should know the patient's recent blood glucose trends when calling an endocrinologist for assistance with diabetes management.

Specific Question

Few consultants like to hear the phrase, "We don't know what's going on and need your help." Try to have a specific question or objective in mind when calling a consult. Doing so helps the consultant focus his or her search and provide the most relevant assistance.

What to Expect

You should expect the consultant to see your patient in a timely manner, within the parameters you set out during your initial call. The consultant will speak with and examine the patient and should leave a note in the chart documenting his or her findings and recommendations. Sometimes, the consultant will leave a brief note stating that he or she has seen the patient and that a full consultation report will follow shortly. If a resident or fellow sees the patient first, final recommendations may be delayed until the attending consultant has seen the patient as well.

Most consultants will not directly order tests for your patient, and no consultant should change your orders or write new ones without speaking to you first. Some may call you to discuss their findings and recommendations, whereas others leave it to you to read their note in the chart. Make sure you check your patients' charts frequently to look for consultant recommendations. It is acceptable to ask your consultant ahead of time to order any tests he or she deems appropriate. If you disagree with a consultant's findings and do not plan on implementing the recommendations, you should call to discuss the matter directly.

Communication after the Initial Consult

Unless your specific question has been answered fully at the first visit, the consultant should return to see the patient. Some patients necessitate daily visits from your consultant, whereas others can be seen less frequently. *Again, make sure to check the chart daily for new recommendations.*

Consultant Signing Off

Most consultants will leave a brief "sign-off" note in the chart when they feel their services are no longer required. If you disagree, don't hesitate to call and discuss the matter with the consultant directly. If you have not seen a recent note from the consultant and no "sign-off" note was entered, call to find out if he or she plans continued participation in the patient's care.

DISCHARGES

Discharged patients are usually eager to get out of the hospital. Thus:

- Have the paperwork for discharges finished as soon as possible after rounds. You can even prepare some of it the day before.

- Make sure that the other services involved in the patient's care are notified so they can provide final recommendations and schedule follow-up appointments.

- Ask the patient if he or she would like you to call any family members for them. Families are frequently overwhelmed when a patient is sent home while still in the recovery phase. Make sure you take time to answer their questions about diet, pain pills, exercise, and follow-up appointments. Let them know what to expect and what warrants a call to the surgeon's office.

See also Chap. 5, Discharges.

ADMISSIONS AND TRANSFERS

In addition to postoperative patients, you will receive three types of new patients: admissions from the ER, transfers from outside hospitals, and scheduled admissions for preoperative evaluation. Your role in the workup of these patients will vary depending on how extensive an evaluation they have already received.

- See all new patients on their arrival to the floor. Make sure the appropriate diagnostic testing is under way.

- It is wise to review the case with your senior or attending as soon as possible. Prompt communication prevents any delay in workup or treatment.

- Waiting until evening rounds to review the case is acceptable for the stable patient with a known diagnosis but riskier in an ill patient or one with an unclear diagnosis.

LABS AND X-RAYS

- Review the lab data from each of your patients during the early part of the day so you can act on anything abnormal. Waiting until 3 p.m. to learn that the CBC drawn at 5 a.m. showed a hematocrit of 24 is not good for you or your patient. Record the data on your list so you have the numbers available on evening rounds. Follow up on any labs ordered on morning rounds.

- It is also important to check your patients' microbiology results daily.

- Any x-rays pending should be sought out early.

• If your patient requires preparation for a CT scan or other imaging (e.g., NPO, drinking contrast), you should make sure it's under way so the scan will not be delayed (see Chap. 20, Contrast Agents).

CHART REVIEW

It is good practice to review the chart at some point before evening rounds. You will find important notes from consultants, therapists, and nurses. This information will help you plan the care of your patients. In addition, asking for a consultation and then not following the recommendations in a timely fashion will not win you any friends.

GETTING TO THE OR

Your ability to spend time in the OR is program specific. If you are given the opportunity, take advantage of it, even if it means staying later in the evening to finish up the floor work.

POSTOPERATIVE CHECKS

It will be important for you to know what patients to expect to come from the OR.

• Review the OR schedule each morning.

• When a nurse calls to notify you of a patient's arrival, it is best to see the patient briefly at that time. You play an important role in making sure that the postoperative patient is doing well.

• Check on pain control; if it is inadequate, make sure the problem is remedied as quickly as possible.

• You will need to visit all postoperative patients several hours after arrival for the formal postoperative check (see Chap. 18, Postoperative Check).

EVENING ROUNDS

In most programs, your team will round a second time in the afternoon or evening, after the senior residents are finished in the OR. You will be expected to provide brief updates on the progress of each patient, any new data available (labs, x-rays, consults), and descriptions of new problems that arose over the course of the day. In addition, the team is interested in seeing the new postoperative patients to make sure they are recovering as expected.

On evening rounds, the goal is to address new issues that arose during the day and identify potential problems that may occur overnight. In addition, it's the time to decide what orders need to be written for the night nurses. This will usually include morning labs and x-rays.

• You will be much more effective on evening rounds if you have gathered your thoughts beforehand. The best strategy is to make sure all the to-dos from the morning have been done and that you have all lab and x-ray data available on the list.

- Stopping by to check on each patient during the afternoon helps you detect and begin to solve any new problems before the team arrives to see the patients.

- You usually will not need to remake a list for evening rounds, but all new data must be readily available.

- If a patient's diet is to be advanced at breakfast, order it during evening rounds.

- Ordering CT scans and other radiologic testing ahead of time is also advantageous.

AFTER EVENING ROUNDS

After you finish rounding with the team, begin working on the tasks generated during evening rounds.

- Obtain the office charts of patients to be admitted the next day.

- Before signing out, make sure you have finished everything that can be done at that time.

- Check on the results of any acute interventions you made on evening rounds (e.g., urine output response to a fluid bolus, appropriate pain control after changing to patient-controlled analgesia).

SIGNING OUT

There are many ways of signing out to the on-call intern, but it is always helpful to provide a copy of the updated list.

- You must include all new patients (admissions, transfers, postoperatives).

- List any things remaining to check on and approximate times that they should be done. For example, if you ask someone to check on a CBC, you should know if it has already been drawn and when the result should be expected.

- Identify the sickest patients, who will need to be monitored closely.

- Prepare all of the above in a legible and organized fashion.

- Finally, provide the telephone or beeper numbers of the appropriate senior residents to call with problems.

HEADING HOME

By the time you sign out to the covering team, you have had a long and busy day. When the time comes to go home, don't hang around the hospital. You will be a much happier and more effective intern if you find some time for yourself during the year.

- Plan what free time you have very carefully, and closely guard the little daylight you will see.

- Spend some time doing whatever makes you feel human. Exercise outside, call friends and family, hang out at a coffee shop with a fellow intern, or fix a home-cooked meal.

- Schedule some time for reading as well. This can be done at home and may also be incorporated into your call night.

3

Call Night

Emily R. Winslow

For most new surgical interns, the call night is approached with some trepidation. There is no question that being on call can, at times, be laborious and stressful. At other times, it is equally exhilarating, challenging, and rewarding.

During the day, many people are in the hospital to help with any situation. At night, fewer people are available. You will have some independence and be able to solve familiar problems on your own, but you may be put in situations that you are not familiar with and may feel as if you are alone in managing some very sick patients. The most important piece of advice about being on call is to *know whom to call for help and when*. There is no such thing as a stupid question when the answer could affect a patient's course. You will find that many people are willing to hear from you in the middle of the night. *Always call for help when you need it*. Remember that no surgeon wants to learn about a serious problem with his or her patient 8 hrs after it started. Effective communication on your part means that your senior resident or attending will have no surprises during morning rounds. Here are some important things to build into your call night routine.

SIGN OUT

Transferring critical information efficiently and correctly from one person to another is at the heart of the sign out process. Your job as the intern on call is to get sign out from the other interns before they leave the hospital (see Chap. 2, Organizing Your Day).

CALLS FROM THE NURSE

Answering calls from nursing personnel about any number of problems will constitute the majority of your call night. For common call night questions, see Part V, Common Calls.

SCHEDULED CHECKS ON SICK PATIENTS

Recognize that not all problems will be noted by the nursing staff in a timely fashion. If you know of a patient who is particularly ill or is not doing well, plan to visit that patient several times throughout the evening to see how things are progressing. Often, the covering team avoids these sicker patients, because their problems seem complex and their courses are unfamiliar. *Do not fall into the trap of avoiding these patients until you are called about them.* You will provide better patient care and learn more about surgical patients if you make a point of being closely involved with their management.

INTERN ROUNDS

Although rounds are normally thought of as a team activity, one helpful strategy for dealing with patients while on call is to make solo rounds at night. This is best done around 9–10 p.m., while patients are still awake. Taking the time to round on your own has several benefits:

1. **You will pick up on any developing problems early in their course.** For example, getting on top of pain early is much easier and kinder than waiting until the patient is in significant distress.
2. **You will be able to avoid many routine calls.** By checking on patients and asking about any problems, you will be better equipped to handle issues that come up later in the night. Patients may ask for sleeping pills or a change in pain medicine, issues that are more easily addressed at 10 p.m. than at 3 a.m.
3. **You will learn the typical postoperative course.** Seeing numerous patients throughout their hospital stay is the best way for you to learn what the expected postoperative course is. You will benefit from even a brief visit.
4. **Patients appreciate being seen by the doctor.** In a large teaching hospital, patients are often troubled by the number of doctors taking care of them. However, when they begin to realize that the on-call doctor takes individual interest in them, they will be happier and more trusting.
5. **You will develop a rapport with the nurses.** Checking in with nurses before you head to your call room enables you to address any of their concerns and lets them know that you are part of "the team."

GETTING TO THE OR

One of the benefits of staying in the hospital overnight is the possibility of being involved in an emergency case. This may mean a case that you will get to do, such as an appendectomy, or a complex trauma case that you may only get to observe. Either way, it is a good learning experience for you to be in the OR.

READING

Depending on your patient load, you may find yourself with free time while on call. If this happens, you can take advantage of it by reading. One effective strategy is to keep a few pages of reading material in your pocket—far less cumbersome than carrying a textbook, and you are more likely to read it during a few moments of downtime. Many reference materials are now also available in an electronic format to keep on your PDA.

SLEEPING

You may be lucky enough to get some sleep while on call. Do several important things before going to bed:

- Check in with each nursing station and make sure they know the number to the call room where you will be in case you do not answer your page. Eager but sleep-deprived interns sometimes sleep through their pages.

- Remember to set an alarm or get a wake-up call early enough to meet with the other interns who signed out to you.

- Most important, expect to be woken frequently, and expect to leave your bed to see your patients.

4

Talking to Families

Emily R. Winslow

. . . no, Mrs. Jones, I would not like to date your single, unattached daughter/son . . .

Although you may not have had any formal instruction on the subject of talking to families during medical school, it is one of the more important skills to have as a resident. There is no such thing as "routine" surgery to a patient or patient's family members. Close friends' and relatives' lives change significantly when one of their loved ones is in the hospital or undergoing surgery. They are anxious, scared, concerned, and confused. Do your best to answer their questions and relieve them of any unnecessary worry. Your patients may not remember your good care, but their families will.

WHO SHOULD DO THE TALKING?

Make an effort to touch base with a patient's family daily. Your role in talking to the family will vary from service to service. Often, your senior resident and attending will be talking to the family primarily and will rely on you when they are not available. Make sure you understand if and when it is your job.

Remember not to get in over your head. If you don't know the data and your attending's opinions, remain silent. Let the family know that you will discuss the issue with the attending. Conflicting information from different members of the team only complicates the situation. Communicating with the patient and family is ultimately the responsibility of the attending. Your attending will often want to be the one to explain the findings and treatment recommendations.

PREOP

Make sure that the family and patient understand the nature of the operation, its indication, and its possible complications.

IMMEDIATELY AFTER THE OPERATION

The family members are usually all gathered from the time a patient is taken into preoperative holding until he or she is released from recovery. This waiting period is difficult for them and they are watching the clock, waiting expectantly for the surgeon's appearance. Any delay suggests to them that a complication has occurred.

It is the attending's job to talk to the family after the case, but it is wise for you to stop by the waiting room after taking the patient to recovery to ensure that the surgeon has been there. If the attending has not yet been by, reassure the family and tell them that they can expect to see the surgeon later. It helps to tell them the range of hours when the attending and team will be making rounds that evening.

ON TRANSFER TO THE ICU

If a patient requires an unexpected trip to the ICU, it is critical to let the family know about it before they arrive at the hospital and find their family member's room empty. The easiest way to notify them is with a phone call at the time of transfer (even if it is the middle of the night). Reassure them as much as possible about the patient's condition and then tell them where and when they will be able to see their family member. (Remember that ICUs have strict visiting hours, and having the family rush to the hospital only to sit in the waiting room is not helpful.)

ON RETURN TO THE OR

If for any reason a patient requires return to the OR, let the family know as far in advance as possible. Again, even the smallest of procedures is not trivial to them.

SIGNIFICANT CHANGE IN CONDITION

Significant change in condition is a much more difficult scenario. Any time a patient's course changes rapidly and for the worse, the family should be informed.

DISCHARGE

Often, family members will be taking care of the postoperative patient on discharge, so it is best to let them know about the discharge as far ahead of time as possible. They will usually have lots of questions about what to do when they get home. Answer them in as much detail as you can; it will save them from having to make unnecessary calls. Make sure they understand when and how to get a follow-up appointment. Let them know exactly whom to get in touch with and how if something goes wrong after hours (see also Chap. 5, Discharges).

5 Discharges

Jeremy Goodman

. . . When can I shower?

Discharge planning begins on the day of admission. Every day, you should consider whether each patient is ready to go home. Plan far enough in advance so that on the day of discharge, everything has been set up for a smooth transition out of the hospital.

PRESCRIPTIONS
Make sure the patient is discharged with prescriptions for any new medications.

- The names, dosages, and instructions for use should be included on a discharge sheet. Be sure to specify if the patient is to stop taking a previously prescribed medication.

- Include the hospital or switchboard operator phone number on all prescriptions. Don't include your personal pager number on the paperwork.

- Review the patient's medical record for narcotic needs. You must provide a sufficient quantity of analgesics to ensure that the patient will be comfortable at home. If you do not have a license to prescribe narcotics, remember to have a senior resident sign the prescription. Don't wait until everyone has gone to the OR for the day, as doing so will unnecessarily delay your patient's discharge. Virtually all patients who are discharged with narcotics will benefit from the addition of a stool softener. It should be taken as long as the narcotics continue to be used.

- Ask if the patient needs prescriptions for home (preoperative) medications.

HOME NEEDS
As hospital length of stay has decreased over the years, more patients are being discharged home with allied health professional assistance. This includes home or outpatient physical and occupational therapy visits, skilled nursing, and social work. Many hospitals have case coordinators or discharge planners to help with the details. Get into the habit of reviewing your patient census with the planners daily. Make sure all necessary services are in place before the patient is discharged.

- Patients discharged with open wounds require dressing changes.

- Those with indwelling central lines, drains, and TPN should have home health nursing visits arranged.

- Some patients require supplemental oxygen, either temporarily or permanently, after discharge. Strict criteria need to be met for approval of home oxygen and reimbursement of the expense. Assessment usually involves resting and exercise pulse oximetry. If you anticipate a patient's need for continued oxygen therapy, arrange for testing on the day before discharge, and ensure that both a portable transport tank and home unit are available.

ACTIVITY LEVEL

You may wish to limit your patient's activities after certain operations.

- After laparotomy, 4 wks of light activities without heavy lifting are generally recommended.

- Patients who have undergone extremity or peripheral vascular surgery should keep the affected limb elevated to reduce swelling.

- Limitations to activity are procedure specific. Check with your attending.

INCISION CARE

- Most wounds can be wet after 48 hrs but not soaked in a tub or pool.

- Scar tissue is very sensitive to sunburn, and patients should be encouraged to use sunscreen on incisions that will be exposed to the sun. They should wait 1–2 wks before applying any lotions to a new incision.

RETURN VISIT

Check with each attending regarding the return visit policy.

- Thoracic, abdominal, and extremity staples and sutures are usually removed in 7–10 days. Facial and neck sutures are removed sooner.

- Patients discharged with an indwelling drain should keep a daily log of outputs and bring it to the first office visit.

EXTENDED CARE FACILITIES AND TRANSFERS

Not all discharges will find the patient going directly home. Sometimes, patients will be transferred to another hospital where specialized services or a particular physician is available.

- For interhospital transfers, you should prepare a concise summary of the patient's recent course and include copies of relevant paperwork and imaging studies.

- Transfers to a nursing home, extended care facility, or rehabilitation center should also include a hospital summary. These facilities usually require transfer orders, including medications, diet, activities, and specific nursing responsibilities, such as wound care.

- When possible, include a copy of the dictated discharge summary (if your hospital uses a dictation system). Dictating the summary the day before will help to ensure that it has been transcribed in time for the transfer (see Appendix B, Common Templates).

REMOVAL OF LINES, TUBES, AND DRAINS

Most patients are not sent home with indwelling IV lines and drains. Make sure these are removed before discharge.

- In some hospitals, nurses can remove central venous catheters or surgical drains, but remember that it is ultimately your responsibility to ensure that it has been done.

- Patients should remain in bed for at least 30 mins after central venous catheter removal.

- Patients should not be discharged from the hospital after removal of a urinary catheter until they have voided.

DICTATION

Most hospitals require a dictated discharge summary for record keeping and billing purposes. Responsibility for completion usually falls on the intern.

- Essential components of the discharge summary include
  - attending surgeon's name
  - dates of admission and discharge
  - diagnoses
  - procedures performed
  - brief summary of the patient's medical history, presenting physical exam, and pertinent studies
  - hospital course
  - discharge instructions

- You do not need to describe the routine facets of the patient's postoperative recovery. Include the indications for, and results of, all significant studies performed.

- Discuss the hospital course in a problem-focused way. Your discharge summary should enable the next physician taking care of this patient to quickly understand the significance of the patient's hospital visit.

- Get into the habit of completing summaries as soon as the patient is discharged; dictations have a way of piling up otherwise.

6 Against Medical Advice

Jeremy Goodman

. . . if left untreated, that ingrown toenail could KILL you!

Despite your best intentions, you will occasionally encounter the patient who does not wish further medical care. This is more common in the trauma population. Remember that unless the patient is unable to fully comprehend the consequences of his or her actions (e.g., in intoxication or dementia), you have no right to detain him or her. Psychiatric patients being legally held as a danger to themselves or others are a different category.

- If a patient wishes to leave the hospital against medical advice, first confirm that the patient is alert, oriented, and competent. Competence is difficult to define and can be even harder to assess. Consider asking for a psychiatry consult if there is any question.

- Explain in detail exactly what care you would like to deliver and the potential consequences of refusal. Make it clear that the patient may change his or her mind at any time and return for further treatment.

- Have a nurse or other health professional witness your discussion.

- Most institutions have a form for the patient to sign that acknowledges the discussion and relieves the team and hospital of liability. Ask the patient to carefully read and sign the form; understand that some patients may refuse to sign.

- In any case, fully document the events in the medical record, and of course notify your senior resident and attending as soon as possible.

- A related event is patient elopement. Some patients will decide against treatment and leave the hospital before you can be summoned. As above, fully document the scenario in the medical record and make sure the nurses do the same.

7

Expirations

Jeremy Goodman

. . . transfer to the eternal care unit . . .

As hard as we try to save every patient, some are truly beyond our reach. Patient deaths may be anticipated or unexpected and are always emotionally trying. Remember, many people are involved in a patient's care, and concerned family members may be far from the hospital. Your responsibility is to inform these people in a timely fashion and complete any paperwork required by your institution. This chapter deals with such details; aspects of resuscitation and running a code are discussed in Part VII, Critical Care.

CALLS TO MAKE

- **Senior resident:** Immediately inform your senior resident of a patient's expiration.

- **Attending:** Check with your senior on who should call the attending. Some senior residents prefer to do this themselves. Several attending surgeons often are involved in a patient's care, and all need to be informed.

- **Family:** This is probably the most difficult task, and it will sometimes fall to you. It is also the most important and should never be overlooked. Be prepared for a wide range of reactions, from breathless silence to anguished weeping. Your announcement will be taken much worse if unexpected, underscoring the need for frequent and honest communication with all families, especially those of your sickest patients.

  - You should ask about an autopsy in virtually all cases. An autopsy answers important questions about the cause of death and can help educate the surgery team. While you may gently encourage an autopsy, you should never force it on a family. Be sure to explain that such an exam will not interfere with funeral home or burial arrangements and that the incisions cannot be seen. Some families will agree to a limited autopsy excluding certain areas, such as the head. Whatever the family's decision, it should be accepted and respected. A specific set of criteria defines coroner's cases requiring a postmortem exam by the local medical examiner.

- Many patients are candidates for anatomic gifts, including whole organ donation for transplant as well as tissue donation. If you anticipate that a patient is a donor candidate, get the local organ procurement organization involved early. Their trained counselors specialize in talking to families about anatomic gifts.

PAPERWORK

Each institution has its own set of papers to fill out for patient expirations.

- Often, you will be asked to fill out a preliminary death certificate. This form requires the proximate cause of death; "cardiac arrest" is not an acceptable answer. Include the disease process or processes that contributed to the patient's death. Remember that what you write has significant medicolegal implications. If you are unsure, ask your senior resident for help.

- Documentation in the chart is a must. Write a note describing the patient's condition on your arrival and that death was confirmed (i.e., absence of heartbeat on auscultation or asystole on ECG). Include the time of death and document those people you informed (attending, family).

- Many hospitals also require a dictated expiration note. Although similar in form to the dictated discharge summary, it does not need to be as lengthy or detailed. Include a brief description of the patient's presentation, procedures, hospital course, and events leading up to the death.

Resources

8 Books

Jeremy Goodman,
Nirmal K. Veeramachaneni,
and Emily R. Winslow

. . . you can call on me . . .

Baker RJ, Fischer JE. *Mastery of surgery*, 2nd ed. Philadelphia: Lippincott Williams & Wilkins, 2001.

Berger DH, Feig BW, Fuhrman G, eds. *The M.D. Anderson surgical oncology handbook*, 2nd ed. Philadelphia: Lippincott Williams & Wilkins, 1998.

Blackbourne LH, ed. *Surgical recall*. Philadelphia: Lippincott Williams & Wilkins, 1998.

Cameron JL. *Current surgical therapy*, 7th ed. St. Louis: Mosby, 2001.

Corson JD, Williamson RCN, eds. *Surgery*. St. Louis: Mosby, 2001.

Doherty GM, Meko JB, Olson JA, et al., eds. *The Washington manual of surgery*, 2nd ed. Philadelphia: Lippincott Williams & Wilkins, 1999.

Greenfield LJ, Mulholland MW, Oldham K. *Surgery: scientific principles and practice*, 3rd ed. Philadelphia: Lippincott Williams & Wilkins, 2001.

Lawrence PF. *Essentials of general surgery*, 3rd ed. Philadelphia: Lippincott Williams & Wilkins, 2000.

Norton JA, Bollinger RR, Lowry SF, et al., eds. *Surgery: basic science and clinical evidence*. New York: Springer-Verlag, 2000.

Schwartz SI, Galloway AC, Shires T, eds. *Principles of surgery*, 7th ed. New York: McGraw-Hill, 1998.

Townsend CM, Beauchamp DR, eds. *Sabiston textbook of surgery: the biological basis of modern surgical practice*, 16th ed. Philadelphia: WB Saunders, 2001.

Zollinger RM. *Atlas of surgical operations*, 7th ed. New York: McGraw-Hill, 1997.

9

Internet Resources

**Jeremy Goodman,
Nirmal K. Veeramachaneni,
and Emily R. Winslow**

JOURNALS

jama.ama-assn.org (Journal of the American Medical Association)
ats.ctsnetjournals.org (Annals of Thoracic Surgery)
link.springer.de/link/service/journals/10016/index.htm (Annals of Vascular Surgery)
archsurg.ama-assn.org (Archives of Surgery)
www.journalacs.org (Journal of the American College of Surgeons)
www.otago.ac.nz/surgery/1journals.html (WWW Surgical Journals Status)
www.harcourthealth.com/periodicals (Various journals)
www.nejm.org (New England Journal of Medicine)

ORGANIZATIONS

www.ama-assn.org (American Medical Association)
www.aast.org (American Association for the Surgery of Trauma)
www.abcrs.org (American Board of Colon and Rectal Surgery)
www.facs.org (American College of Surgeons)
www.asbs.org (American Society for Bariatric Surgery)
www.breastsurgeons.org (American Society of Breast Surgeons)
www.fascrs.org (American Society of Colon and Rectal Surgeons)
www.asts.org (American Society of Transplant Surgeons)
www.womensurgeons.org (Association of Women Surgeons)
ics-us.org (International College of Surgeons)
www.ssat.com (Society for Surgery of the Alimentary Tract)
www.sages.org (Society of American Gastrointestinal Endoscopic Surgeons)
www.sls.org (Society of Laparoendoscopic Surgeons)
www.sts.org (Society of Thoracic Surgery)
www.east.org (Eastern Association for the Surgery of Trauma)
www.unos.org (United Network for Organ Sharing)

ONCOLOGY

www.nci.nih.gov (National Cancer Institute)
www.surgical-oncology.net (Surgical Oncology Net)

REFERENCES

www.mdconsult.com (online journals and texts)
www.ncbi.nlm.nih.gov/PubMed (Medline)
www.merckmedicus.com (Merck Medicus)

Perioperative Care and Conduct

10

Preoperative Cardiac Assessment

Ravi Gurujal

. . . I smoke, eat hot wings, and don't exercise. What's my risk, doc?

RISK STRATIFICATION

Cardiac morbidity is an enormous problem in surgical patients. An estimated 50% of perioperative mortality is cardiac in etiology. Moreover, perioperative cardiac morbidity leads to poor long-term outcome; evidence of ischemia on Holter monitor in the first postoperative 48 hrs is associated with a doubling of mortality at 2 yrs. The 6-mo prognosis in patients with a diagnosis of postoperative myocardial infarction (MI) is dismal, with mortality as high as 50–70%. Even though your patients may have been cleared for surgery preoperatively, you should have a clear understanding of cardiac risk stratification.

The American College of Cardiology has designed a paradigm through which these problems can be minimized. This chapter introduces these guidelines in a stepwise fashion and provides a brief explanation of each step's rationale.

Three central questions form the basis of risk stratification:

1. **What is the cardiac history, and are there any cardiac symptoms?**
2. **What is the patient's exercise tolerance?**
3. **What is the intrinsic risk of the proposed surgery?**

The answers, along with the results of an ECG, lead to a course of action that allows one to minimize the risk of postoperative MI.

STEP 1: IDENTIFY EMERGENCY PROCEDURES (PART OF CENTRAL QUESTION 3)

By definition, an emergent procedure takes precedence over any further cardiac evaluation. Emergency operations increase the risk of cardiac complications, and patients should be managed with perioperative beta-blockade if the clinical condition permits.

STEP 2: IDENTIFY THE CARDIAC-REVASCULARIZED PATIENT (PART OF CENTRAL QUESTION 1)

Patients who have undergone cardiac revascularization (coronary artery bypass grafting, percutaneous transluminal coronary angioplasty, stents) within the last 5 yrs and have good exercise tolerance (see step 6 below) without recurrent symptoms have operative cardiac morbidity lower than the unselected general population.

STEP 3: REVIEW ANY RECENT CARDIAC EVALUATION (PART OF CENTRAL QUESTION 1)

Obtain the results of recent ECGs, stress tests, echocardiograms, and angiograms.

STEPS 4 AND 5: IDENTIFY THE PATIENT'S CLINICAL RISK AND ORDER NECESSARY DIAGNOSTIC TESTS (PART OF CENTRAL QUESTION 1)

The clinical risk assessment is an extremely important part of the preoperative evaluation, both for prognosis and to guide further testing.

The most important task (step 4) is to identify those patients with *unstable angina, decompensated congestive heart failure (CHF), recent MI, hemodynamically significant arrhythmias, or critical valve diseases*. These patients are at very high risk and should have nonemergent surgeries deferred.

Treatment decisions for patients with unstable angina, hemodynamically significant arrhythmias, or decompensated CHF should be made in conjunction with a cardiologist. It is prudent to wait 4–6 wks after a documented MI to proceed with elective surgery. Very severe aortic stenosis (AS) with a valve area <0.75 cm^2 or symptomatic AS should still be considered a high-risk condition.

For other patients, various indices have been created and validated that separate patients into low- and intermediate-risk populations. The most famous is the Goldman index. The number of risk factors and the varying points assigned per factor make many such indices cumbersome for daily use. Some risk factors that have been shown in multivariate analyses to have independent predictive value for perioperative cardiac morbidity are

- ◆ CHF
- ◆ Diabetes
- ◆ Prior MI
- ◆ Angina
- • Ventricular arrhythmia (treated)
- • Age >70
- • History of stroke
- • Preoperative renal insufficiency (creatinine >2)
- • Poor exercise tolerance
- • AS

- S_3 on exam

- Elevated jugular venous pressure

The current recommendation is for *all patients with any of the first four risk factors (◆) who will undergo high-risk surgery to have noninvasive cardiac testing*. Patients without any of the first eight (or even five) risk factors have such a low event rate that testing will likely only generate false-positives unless they have very poor exercise tolerance. However, keep in mind that these are only guidelines. If you believe that your patient is at higher-than-average risk for any reason, it is prudent to order some preoperative cardiac testing. Consult a cardiologist; it is always in the patient's best interest to be sure of the appropriate course of action.

There is evidence that beta-blocked patients with two or fewer of the first eight risk factors can be managed without stress testing. Beta-blockers reduce MI risk to nearly the same levels of patients who undergo coronary bypass grafting before their noncardiac surgery. Bottom line: *Beta-blockers are essential for all high-risk patients and all patients undergoing high-risk surgery*.

A number of protocols have been used to initiate beta-blockers. If the patient is normally on these medications, remember to continue them. One protocol is especially salient to the surgeon and should be discussed with the anesthesiologist:

- If the heart rate is >55 BPM, the systolic BP is >100 mm Hg, and there is no evidence of CHF, third-degree heart block, or bronchospasm, 5 mg of IV atenolol (Tenormin) may be infused over a period of 5 mins starting 30 mins before entry into the OR.

- The patient is observed for an additional 5 mins, and if the above criteria continue to be met, another 5-mg dose is given.

- Immediately after surgery, a 5-mg dose is given in the same way.

- Starting on the morning of the first postoperative day, and continuing until discharge, the patient receives either 5 mg of IV atenolol (q12h) or PO atenolol qd; 100 mg if the heart rate is >65 BPM and the systolic BP is >100 mm Hg; 50 mg if the heart rate is >55 but <65 and the systolic BP is >100 mm Hg.

- No atenolol should be given if the heart rate is <55, the systolic BP is <100 mm Hg, or there is evidence of CHF or bronchospasm.

As always, speak with your senior resident before initiating such therapy.

STEP 6: IDENTIFY EXERCISE TOLERANCE (CENTRAL QUESTION 2)

Formal exercise stress testing and history are used to identify exercise tolerance. Patients who cannot walk four blocks on level ground or up two flights of stairs have a cardiac event rate that is approximately twice that of patients able to complete these tasks. Many patients don't know their exercise tolerance and will overestimate it. You must have a high degree of confidence in a patient's assessment of his or her abilities before canceling a stress test that would otherwise be indicated.

STEP 7: IDENTIFY THE RISK OF SURGERY (CENTRAL QUESTION 3)

Noncardiac operations can be divided into high-, intermediate-, and low-risk procedures. The risk of surgery appears to be intrinsic to the procedure and not necessarily to the type of anesthesia; in other words, epidural anesthesia does not seem to have a lower cardiovascular morbidity than does general anesthesia. The categories of risk can be blurred depending on the study, but a general stratification is listed below. One salient point is that *emergent operations are consistently riskier than the same procedure performed electively; any high- or intermediate-risk operation that is done emergently should probably be managed with perioperative beta-blockade unless contraindications exist.* Lengthy procedures and significant blood loss lead to increased risk.

High-Risk Procedures

Death or MI (>4%) in patient with medically treated coronary artery disease

- Noncarotid vascular surgery

- Thoracic procedures

- Abdominal procedures

- Major head and neck procedures

- Any emergent surgery

Intermediate-Risk Procedures

Death or MI (1–4%)

- Carotid surgery

- Radical prostatectomy

- Orthopedic procedures

Low-Risk Procedures

Death or MI (<1%)

- Ophthalmologic procedures

- Transurethral prostate resection

- Breast surgery

- Biopsies

- Minor head and neck procedures

STEP 8: ORDER NONINVASIVE TESTING FOR APPROPRIATE PATIENTS

The American College of Cardiology guidelines recommend noninvasive testing for two groups of patients: (a) anyone with poor exercise tolerance undergoing a high-risk procedure and (b) any patient with intermediate clinical risk and poor exercise tolerance undergoing intermediate-risk surgery.

There are no general rules on the type of stress test (stress echocardiogram or chemically stressed nuclear imaging) that should be ordered; each test gives slightly different diagnostic and prognostic information.

- Echocardiography appears to be slightly more specific but less sensitive. Stress echoes do have the advantage of providing other anatomic information, such as valve detail.

- Nuclear imaging has the advantage of being easier to perform on the patient with a large body habitus and is less operator dependent.

- Remember, both tests are most useful when they are normal (a fixed defect or resting wall motion abnormality is not normal) or when there is no evidence of ischemia.

- Note that for a given amount of ischemia, diabetics seem to have double the risk.

Even if the stress test comes back positive, a certain percentage of patients can be managed with perioperative beta-blockade alone. The decision should be made in conjunction with a cardiologist. Many patients will be considered for coronary angiography and subsequent revascularization. To benefit the patient, the combined risk of revascularization with subsequent surgery has to be less than the risk of the proposed surgery combined with the long-term risk of nonrevascularized coronary artery disease.

CONCLUSION

In the cardiac preoperative assessment, remember to ask the following questions:

- Have you ever had a heart attack or surgery for your heart?

- Have you ever had any testing on your heart (stress test, echo, cath)?

- Do you ever have chest pain or shortness of breath, either at rest or on exertion?

- Can you walk four blocks on level ground or up two flights of stairs?

Ask yourself the risk of surgery and order imaging studies as appropriate. Look for Q waves on the ECG.

The accurate assessment of cardiac risk factors can go a long way toward avoiding postoperative morbidity and mortality. When in doubt, ask a cardiologist for assistance.

11

Preoperative Blood Work and Imaging

Nirmal K. Veeramachaneni

Most interns have a tendency to draw too many preoperative labs. Remember that a lab value is of no significance if it *does not change your management*.

- From the surgeon's perspective, some studies are clearly indicated. For example, infection is a concern when implanting a foreign object, such as a graft or pacemaker, so you should rule out an occult UTI that could seed the implanted object.

- Apart from such surgical issues and disease-specific needs, little is required for the anesthesiologists' purposes. Always check with a senior resident for your institution's policies. Numerous guidelines exist, and Table 11-1 reflects the policy of the Department of Anesthesia at Barnes-Jewish Hospital in St. Louis. A minor procedure is a short one in which little or no blood loss is expected, whereas a major procedure is one in which potential for blood loss exists.

- The ECG, chest x-ray, and blood studies are acceptable within 6 mos of the date of surgery if there have been no interim changes in the medical condition or treatment of the patient. Some tests, such as glucose, blood bank (type and screen), and electrolyte assessment in the renal patient, should be done much closer to the time of surgery.

- Tumor markers may, in some patients, be drawn preoperatively as a baseline to help in the later detection of recurrence.

- Comorbid conditions and medications influence what lab testing is indicated. Patients with stable heart disease or peripheral vascular disease need an ECG within 6 mos of surgery. A chest x-ray is indicated when there is a suspicion of congestive heart failure and in patients with pulmonary disease; a new chest x-ray is required if there has been a change in pulmonary status. *From a practical standpoint, essentially all patients with cardiovascular disease or pulmonary disease need both a chest x-ray and ECG in the immediate preoperative period.*

- Numerous other studies, including imaging, are done for surgical procedures. It usually is your job to make sure that these studies are available in the OR. There is nothing worse than finding a mass in the liver on palpation and not having the abdominal CT scan with which to correlate. For a given procedure, make sure you have the right image! Usually, numerous films are kept in the patient's x-ray jacket. Look at the films yourself, and make sure you have the appropriate studies before the patient goes to the OR.

TABLE 11-1.
PREOPERATIVE TESTING: MINIMUM RECOMMENDATIONS

	Type and screen	Hematocrit	Platelets	INR	PTT	Glucose	Potassium	Creatinine	Chest x-ray	ECG
Procedure										
Minor										
Major	x	x								
Age										
<6 mos		x								
>50 yrs										x
Associated conditions										
Cardiovascular									x	x
Pulmonary									x	
Liver			x	x						
Renal							x	x		
Diabetes						x		x		x
Bleeding disorder			x	x	x					
Medications										
Diuretics							x			
Digitalis							x			
Coumadin				x						
Heparin					x					
Pregnancy	All patients who could be pregnant should have beta-hCG levels measured on day of surgery (i.e., women of child-bearing age)									

12 Bowel Prep

Nirmal K. Veeramachaneni

. . . when all else fails, tap water enemas until clear . . .

A combination of mechanical bowel prep (GoLYTELY, Fleet's phospho-soda, or enemas) with antibiotics [a combination of oral neomycin (Mycifradin) and metronidazole (Flagyl)] decreases bacterial load and risk of infection from bowel surgery. A suggested protocol consists of an antibiotic and mechanical bowel regimen:

- Clear liquid diet, NPO after midnight before surgery.
- Fleet's phosphosoda, 45 mL PO, on arrival to ward (day before surgery), and repeat once after 6 hrs. Take each dose with 24 oz of water

or

- In patients with cardiac and renal abnormalities, polyethylene glycol (GoLYTELY), 4 L PO

Medications on the day before surgery consist of

- Neomycin (Mycifradin), 1 g PO, at 1200, 1300, and 2200 on the day before surgery (if surgery scheduled for after 1100 the next day, change time to 1600, 1700, and 0200)

and

- Metronidazole (Flagyl), 500 mg PO, at 1200 and 1800 (if surgery scheduled for after 1100 the next day, change time to 1600 and 2200)

13 Preoperative Diet

Nirmal K. Veeramachaneni

To prevent vomiting and aspiration during anesthesia induction, it is important to ensure that the patient has a completely empty stomach before surgery.

- Gastric emptying is influenced by multiple factors. For example, diabetes and pregnancy are associated with decreased emptying.

- A minimum of 6 hrs should elapse between the ingestion of solids and time of surgery. Although the anesthesia department will usually permit up to 12 oz of clear liquids to be taken up until 2 hrs before the time of surgery, it is general practice to have the patient be entirely NPO after midnight before surgery. This practice ensures there is no miscommunication.

- Medications may be taken with a sip of water.

14 Preoperative Antibiotics

Nirmal K. Veeramachaneni

The incidence of surgical wound infections is decreased with antibiotic administration before skin incision. The type of procedure influences specific choices.

- Most cases require coverage of skin flora (*Staphylococcus* and *Streptococcus* species), usually with a first-generation cephalosporin.

- Bowel surgery also mandates coverage against anaerobes and gram-negative flora. An appropriate second-generation cephalosporin accomplishes this.

- The role of prophylactic antibiotics for clean operations not involving prosthetic material implantation remains controversial. Whether they are used usually depends on the opinion of the attending.

- Perioperative antibiotics should ideally be given from 0–30 mins before incision.

15

Preoperative Holding Area

Nirmal K. Veeramachaneni

The days of admitting a patient the night before a scheduled procedure are over. At the close of morning rounds, your pager may call you to the same-day preoperative holding area to evaluate patients who arrive for surgery. Your job is to confirm and recapitulate the preoperative assessment rapidly and efficiently.

- As usual, good planning is the key. Many other physicians have evaluated this patient before you. The attending surgeon has already evaluated this patient, and consultants may have offered their opinions. These records facilitate a rapid evaluation in the preoperative holding area and assist you postoperatively, when the patient may be unable to provide a complete history.

- On a weekly basis, make a point of checking the following week's operative schedule and seeking the help of the attending surgeon's secretary or nurse for a copy of clinical notes. In many institutions, it is standard practice for the surgeon to submit these notes to the preoperative testing center. This is meant to serve as communication between the anesthesiologist and the surgeon.

- Having reviewed the surgeon's preoperative record, your job now consists of answering the following questions:

  - Has the patient been scheduled for the right operation?

  - Does the patient know what operation he or she is to have?

  - Have the appropriate lab studies been done?

  - Is the patient physically ready for surgery?

  - Has the patient's medical status changed since he or she was evaluated in the office?

- After introducing yourself, briefly review the medical history and confirm that nothing has been missed ("By the way, doc, I had a heart attack last month"). Next, perform a focused physical exam.

- You will have the greatest success in your role as junior resident by focusing your attention on findings that could cause either complications or the case to be canceled. You are the last checkpoint to prevent the patient from having an avoidable surgical complication. For example:

- If a patient presents for dialysis access, ensure the potassium level is not 6.8 with ECG changes.

- Before GI surgery, confirm that the necessary bowel prep has been done.

- Make sure the patient has been NPO.

- Most institutions accept histories and physical exams performed within 30 days of surgery. You should ensure completeness, with a summary of key aspects of the physical exam and brief documentation of new findings. Remember to refer to the existing history and physical if you are not writing a new one.

- If a consent form was not signed at the preoperative office visit, make sure to complete this final task. The consent process is covered in detail in Chap. 16, Consent.

16

Consent

Nirmal K. Veeramachaneni

Consent is not just a signature on a piece of paper. Its purpose is to document that a meaningful conversation has taken place between the patient and surgeon. As junior resident, you will often be the one obtaining informed consent.

- In the conversation with patients, you should answer their questions and address their concerns. If you do not have the answer, do not make one up; defer to your attending or senior resident.

- When possible, involve family members in the discussion.

- Patients should have a realistic understanding of potential outcomes, but it does not need to include a complete list of every possible complication.

- Confirm and then document that a discussion has taken place. A reasonable practice is to make sure that the patient has a good understanding of the procedure, feels all questions have been answered, and wishes to proceed.

- For extremity surgery, specify the side on the consent form.

- For blood consent, always ask patients if they will accept blood products (i.e., find out if they are Jehovah's Witnesses).

- As important as the actual consent form is, it is more important to document in the chart that an informed conversation has taken place.

17

OR Conduct

Nirmal K. Veeramachaneni

. . . don't forget to spin . . .

Finally, you are in your second home! The OR is where you will learn the technical craft of surgery.

Initially, you are expected to learn by watching. Slowly, you will become more involved in the actual procedure. At first, you may do no more than hold tissue out of the way. Remember that your participation is important, no matter how minor it seems. The time will come when you will be supervising your intern through the case.

One way to transition from observer to surgeon is to take an active role in starting the case.

- Timing is everything. You should be in the OR before the attending arrives.

- Introduce yourself to the nursing staff.

- Gather your gown and gloves for the scrub nurse if this has not already been done for you.

- Take off your pager and leave it near the phone. If you forget to do so, the circulating nurse will have to maneuver underneath your gown to retrieve it if it goes off during the case (and it will!).

- You will often be able to speed things along by placing additional IVs or a central line (check with the anesthesia team).

- Learn the principles of airway management, and ask the anesthesiologist if you may intubate the patient. There will inevitably be a time on the ward when you will need these skills emergently.

- Assist in positioning the patient. Proper positioning ensures the prevention of pressure sores, postprocedure muscle pain, and nerve palsies. Furthermore, it permits adequate incision and exposure.

- Place the Foley catheter, shave the surgical field, oversew the ostomy, and do whatever else is needed to perform the operation in an effective and efficient manner. Although the nurse can do most of these tasks, it is your job to ensure they are done properly. When possible, do the task yourself or teach your medical student how to do it.

- Ask if you need to prep the patient. This involves washing the surgical site with an antiseptic solution. It can be done before or after you scrub your hands.

- As you leave the room to scrub your hands, ask if the preoperative antibiotics have been administered (see Chap. 14, Preoperative Antibiotics). Preoperative antibiotics are most effective if administered before the incision is made.

- Finally, never reach for anything on the Mayo stand! The potential for injury exists when more than one person handles sharps.

18 Postoperative Check

Nirmal K. Veeramachaneni

. . . is this supposed to happen after surgery?

The postoperative check is one of the more important responsibilities given to the junior housestaff. Although it can at times seem like merely another box on the checklist to be completed by day's end, it is one of the essential steps in caring for the surgical patient. The goal is to make sure that the patient is not experiencing any postoperative complications.

- For the first 1–2 hrs after surgery, the patient is monitored closely in the recovery room and is then labeled as "stable" and transferred to the regular postoperative floor.

- There are important differences between the patient who is 3 hrs postoperative and the patient who is 3 days postoperative. The former patient is still in a period of significant physiologic stress, whereas the latter has usually reached the point of some physiologic stability.

- First and foremost, *introduce yourself* to your patients and ask them in general how they are doing. You can assess their mental status, pulmonary function, and degree of pain through this short conversation.

- Check the vital signs and note specifically the time of the last measurement. Early postoperative patients need more frequent vital sign measurements than do other patients. Look for the heart rate, BP, respiratory rate, oxygen saturation, and urine output.

- Ask the patient specifically about the following symptoms:

  - **Pain:** It is critical to your therapeutic relationship with the patient that you assess his or her degree of discomfort and act quickly to relieve it as much as possible. You will need to be very sensitive to pain perception so that even if the operation is considered minor, your patient's complaint of pain will not be considered inconsequential.

  - **Chest pain:** Ask about chest pressure, chest discomfort, and chest pain to make sure your patient hasn't experienced myocardial ischemia or infarction during the course of the operation.

- **Shortness of breath:** Check to make sure your patient is oxygenating well and does not have a labored breathing pattern. Remember that pneumothoraces are a possible complication of both assisted ventilation and central line placement, which may have occurred in the OR. Patients with central lines placed in the operating room should always have a postoperative chest x-ray.

- **Nausea and vomiting:** It is common for patients to experience postoperative nausea and vomiting after general anesthesia. You should treat them appropriately with antiemetics, but be cautious of mechanical contributions as well. Patients may require an NG tube for adequate relief of symptoms.

- **Operation-specific complications:** After particular operations, you will need to assess potential complications related to that case. For example, after a carotid endarterectomy, you need to ask about headache, confusion, weakness, numbness, and other signs of neurologic compromise.

- Examine the patient. You should do a focused physical exam. Always listen to the heart and lungs and examine the operative site carefully. Look at the drains and the nature and amount of the output. Postoperative atrial fibrillation, pulmonary edema, and lobar collapse can be diagnosed by a careful physical exam during the postoperative check. Again, for specific operations you will need to perform specific aspects of the exam more carefully. For example, after a lower extremity vascular bypass, you need to feel the temperature of the extremity and carefully assess the pulses. We highlight some key issues to evaluate in Part VI, Common Problems.

- Review the postoperative orders. Usually, they are written by the resident who finished the case. This resident was unable to talk to the patient and therefore may not have written for all necessary home medications. Review the orders for completeness. Make sure the pain, antiemetic, and IV fluid orders are all appropriate to how the patient looks several hours after the operation.

- Look for any postoperative labs or imaging that has been ordered and check to see if they have been completed. Often, this means a CBC and chest x-ray in recovery. You should obtain all results firsthand.

- Think ahead and write any new orders that the patient may need. Some home medications may have been forgotten but will be acceptable for the patient to take. Remember that not all home medications (e.g., anticoagulants, diuretics, and analgesics) should be taken postoperatively. If the patient will need physical therapy, home care, or social work consults, write for those now. If the patient will need lab studies in the morning, they also can be ordered after the postoperative check.

- The postoperative check may be your first chance to meet the patient. In large teaching hospitals, patients are frequently confused as to who the doctor is and what the routine is. Explaining the nature of morning rounds is also helpful, because most patients will not understand why five or six people rush in and out of their room every morning at 6 a.m. Always conclude the postoperative check by asking if the patient has any questions. He or she will usually want to know what the operative findings were (e.g., Was there cancer?). The best way to deal with this is to explain that you were not in the OR and that the attending surgeon will be around later. Do *not* relate findings in the operative note to patients without first talking with your senior resident or attending. Finally, explain the expected trajectory for the next 24–48 hrs. Tell patients if they are NPO, and if so, when they will be able to eat. Tell them what to expect in terms of pain. Tell them about their drains, what purpose they serve, and when they are expected to be removed.

- After you do the above things, you should write a brief postoperative note. If you find anything unexpected, take the appropriate steps to correct the problem immediately. This may mean changing the dose of the patient-controlled analgesia or writing for a chest x-ray, or it may mean notifying a more senior resident of a major postoperative complication.

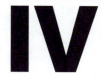 **Radiology and Vascular Studies**

. . . a picture is worth a thousand history and physicals . . .

In this section, we discuss the common tests you may expect to order on a surgical service. Basic indications and interpretation also are reviewed.

19 Communicating with the Radiology Department

Joseph V. Philip

Calling a radiologist is like calling any other consultant. The key pieces of information are

- exam requested
- specific clinical question or clinical situation
- relevant medical diagnoses and surgeries (in cancer patients: last chemotherapy or radiation therapy)
- allergy to iodinated IV dye?
- renal function (serum creatinine)
- IV access: location and gauge
- exam to be portable or in radiology department?
- patient factors, such as size, NPO status, need for mechanical ventilation, and cooperativity

The radiologist may tailor the exam or even suggest a different one to answer the specific clinical question.

Type of IV access is important in studies requiring rapid contrast injection. Most central lines and Port-A-Caths are not large enough to allow rapid contrast injections.

Patient size is an issue when weight is near the table limit or girth precludes entry into the scanner. Some studies are optimal when the patient has been fasting.

20 Contrast Agents

Joseph V. Philip

ORAL CONTRAST

- Barium is usually the GI contrast agent of choice. It should not be used if a leak is suspected or if surgery is imminent, because barium in the peritoneal cavity, although inert, will not reabsorb. Barium can limit future abdominal CT imaging owing to scatter artifact from retained material.

- Water-soluble contrast (Hypaque, Gastroview) is used when barium is contraindicated; however, it produces poorer image quality. It is hyperosmolar and causes fluid shifts into the GI tract (usually not a clinical problem). It should not be used when aspiration is a possibility. In the lungs, it will cause pulmonary edema. Its advantage over barium is that it is reabsorbed from body cavities.

IV CONTRAST
Premedication for Known IV Dye Allergy

- Discuss with the radiologist before initiating any premedication protocol.

- Prednisone (Deltasone), 50 mg PO q6h for three or four doses.

- Some recommend diphenhydramine (Benadryl) just before the exam.

Other IV Contrast Points

- Hold metformin (Glucophage) for 48 hrs after IV contrast administration and check serum creatinine before restarting. The risk is metformin-induced lactic acidosis. Because metformin is primarily cleared by the kidneys, contrast-induced nephropathy may lead to metformin side effects. Holding metformin before the exam is not required.

- Fluid hydration before and after IV contrast can reduce nephrotoxicity. Acetylcysteine (Mucomyst), 600 mg PO bid on the day before and day of IV contrast administration, in conjunction with IV hydration, may decrease nephrotoxicity related to iodinated IV contrast. This benefit has only been shown in patients with chronic renal insufficiency and has not been studied in acute renal failure.

21 Neuroradiology

Joseph V. Philip

NONCONTRAST HEAD CT

- Screening exam for intracranial hemorrhage, increased intracranial pressure, and injury, including fractures.
- Used to follow known intracranial pathology.
- Contrast is useful for evaluation of tumors, although MRI is preferred.

MAGNETIC RESONANCE ANGIOGRAPHY

- Evaluation of circle of Willis and/or neck vessels.
- Conventional angiography is considered the gold standard for evaluation of aneurysms.
- MRI precautions
  - Contraindicated with programmable implanted devices (e.g., pacemakers and cochlear implants), non–MRI-compatible aneurysm clips, and metallic fragments in the eye.
  - Some stents, filters, coils, and prosthetic valves require 6–8 wks to allow tissue ingrowth before an MRI may be performed.
  - MRI compatibility must be considered for other implants, prostheses, metal objects, and some dark tattoos. Closed loop wires have a tendency to heat up during the exam.
  - Skin staples are usually tolerated if secured with tape and gauze.
  - Patients usually must lie flat for 45–90 mins, are unmonitored, and must be cooperative enough to lay still and breath hold. Consider claustrophobia a limitation.

22 **Chest Radiology**

Joseph V. Philip

X-RAY

Pneumothorax (PTX):

- Begin with upright chest x-ray. The classic appearance is a thin, sharp, white line representing the pleural reflection, with air but no vessels beyond the pleura (i.e., air is dark). Skin folds may mimic a PTX but will lack the classic appearance and often extend beyond the chest cavity.

- Also look for a *deep sulcus sign*—lateral costophrenic angle deepening with increased lucency (basilar PTX). Increased lucency over one lung (anterior PTX) or increased sharpness of cardiomediastinal border (medial PTX) is also suggestive.

- Tension PTX: mediastinum shifted away from PTX, hemidiaphragm depressed on side of PTX. In ventilated patients on positive end-expiratory pressure, mediastinal shift may not be present.

CT

- IV contrast for evaluation of great vessels, mediastinum, chest trauma, empyema, and hilar masses.

- Noncontrast CT adequate for evaluating peripheral pulmonary nodules and lung parenchymal disease.

- Pulmonary embolism or aortic dissection protocol: IV contrast is used; a large-bore (18–20 gauge) antecubital IV is required for rapid injection. A central line is not useful for rapid injection.

VENTILATION/PERFUSION (V̇/Q̇) SCAN

- Evaluation of pulmonary embolism

- Performs best when chest x-ray findings are minimal, including no pleural effusions. Recent chest x-ray required

- Good exam for pregnant and young patients (less radiation than CT)

- Can be done at the bedside

PULMONARY ANGIOGRAM

- Evaluation of pulmonary embolism
- Large dye load
- Gold standard

23 Abdominal and Pelvic Radiology

Joseph V. Philip

X-RAY

- Abdomen 1 view is synonymous with KUB (kidneys, ureters, and bladder), AFP (abdominal flat plate), and supine abdomen x-ray.

- Obstructive series: Abdomen 2 view (supine and either upright or left lateral decubitus) and may include an upright chest. The supine film is used to evaluate bowel gas pattern and abnormal calcifications (e.g., renal calculi and appendicoliths), whereas the upright or left lateral decubitus provides the additional evaluation of free intra-peritoneal air and air fluid levels.

  - Normal bowel gas pattern: Nondilated colon with stool and air. Air is also in the rectum. A few loops of nondilated air-filled small bowel are present, as is a gastric bubble. Small bowel folds completely encircle the lumen, and the colonic folds (haustra) only partially encircle the lumen.

  - Complete small bowel obstruction: Most important sign is dilated small bowel. The colon usually has little or no air. Air is usually not seen in the rectum. The more loops of dilated small bowel, the more distal the obstruction.

  - Partial or early small bowel obstruction: Dilated small bowel with some air and stool still seen in the colon and rectum.

  - Ileus: Dilated small and large bowel, with large bowel dilated more prominently than small bowel.

  - Cecal volvulus: Findings of small bowel obstruction and an enlarged cecum that is ectopically located, usually in the left upper quadrant. Should be suspected when an odd left upper quadrant dilated structure is present, as other findings may be subtle.

  - Sigmoid volvulus: Findings of large bowel obstruction (large bowel dilation) and a dilated coffee bean–appearing sigmoid colon (sigmoid folded on itself) in the mid-pelvis.

  - Nonspecific bowel gas pattern: Not normal but not clearly obstructed. Usually a few loops of mildly dilated small bowel or a gasless abdomen. May be seen in many abdominal diseases, such as gastroenteritis or pancreatitis.

- Remember, if dilated loops are fluid filled, they may not be seen. Hence, a paucity of bowel gas may suggest a small bowel obstruction in the appropriate clinical setting.
- Evaluation of free intraperitoneal air:
  - On upright: Subdiaphragmatic air.
  - On left lateral decubitus: Air between liver and body wall. Adequate exam must include the superior liver border/entire right hemidiaphragm.
  - On supine: Often subtle. The inferior liver edge appears sharp; there is increased lucency, especially over the liver; the falciform ligament is outlined by air; the inner and outer margins of bowel wall are well delineated; and there is air not conforming to typical bowel appearance, such as in the subhepatic space.

CT

- Routinely performed with PO and IV contrast.
- The patient is kept NPO except for PO contrast.
- Lack of PO contrast limits the ability to differentiate fluid-filled bowel from loculated fluid collections/abscesses and collapsed bowel from such masses as lymphadenopathy.
- Noncontrast CT (without PO or IV contrast) is used for evaluation of renal stones, retroperitoneal hemorrhage, and aortic aneurysm rupture (routine aortic evaluation is with IV contrast).

ULTRASOUND

- For the evaluation of the liver, gallbladder, bile duct, head of pancreas, kidneys, testicles, ovaries, and uterus.
- May provide guidance for sampling of ascites.
- Fasting required for evaluation of the gallbladder, as it contracts with eating.
- Structures may be obscured by excessive bowel gas.

NUCLEAR MEDICINE
HIDA/DISIDA

- For the evaluation of cholecystitis (including acute, chronic, and acalculous).
- Often used when ultrasound is indeterminate, but can be used as a first-line exam.
- Radiotracer with affinity for excretion into biliary system is injected IV.

- Visualization of the gallbladder in 1 hr excludes cholecystitis. Delayed filling (at >1 hr) suggests chronic cholecystitis. Nonvisualization of the gallbladder is compatible with acute cholecystitis.

GI Bleeding Study

- Used as a screening study for active bleeding to plan immediate intervention.

- Uses radiolabeled (or tagged) RBCs.

- The exam requires drawing a sample of the patient's blood, radiolabeling it, reinjecting (≥30 mins), and 60–90 mins of imaging.

- Sensitivity is 0.1 cc/min of bleeding.

PET

- Radiolabeled tracer (usually glucose) is given IV, and uptake is measured.

- Malignancy usually has a higher glucose metabolism than benign tumors and postoperative scarring.

- Keep patients NPO, hold insulin or PO hypoglycemics before exam, and give no glucose or dextrose in IV fluids.

GI CONTRAST STUDIES
Barium Swallow/Upper GI

- Fluoroscopic exam evaluates esophagus and, if needed, oropharynx.

- Keep the patient NPO.

Small Bowel Follow Through

- Fluoroscopic exam evaluates jejunum and ileum, including terminal ileum.

- Used for Crohn's disease or to rule out small bowel lesions.

- Often performed in conjunction with upper GI exam.

- Keep the patient NPO.

Enteroclysis

- Highly sensitive fluoroscopic evaluation of small bowel.

- Screening often begins with small bowel follow through, because enteroclysis is labor intensive and more uncomfortable.

- Requires that a balloon-tipped, large-bore nasoenteric tube be placed. A bolus of barium is followed by a large volume of methylcellulose to coat and distend the small bowel.

- Keep the patient NPO.

Enema

- Fluoroscopic contrast exam of colon.

- Air contrast (double contrast) exam usually preferred. Initially, colon filled with contrast and subsequently distended with air.

- Excellent mucosal detail.

- Not well tolerated by patients who are not mobile or are generally debilitated. Single contrast exam is performed otherwise. Single contrast exam good for evaluating obstruction, strictures, fistulas, and larger masses.

- Single contrast exam with water-soluble contrast can be performed in the unprepped colon for the additional benefit of cleansing the colon.

- Enema exam usually contraindicated in the setting of active colitis.

- Liquid diet and bowel prep the day before.

OTHER TESTS
IV Pyelogram

- Excellent for evaluating ureters (e.g., for transitional cell carcinoma).

- Series of abdominal x-rays taken after injection of IV contrast.

- Bowel prep the night before to empty overlying colon.

- CT preferred for routine evaluation of renal or ureteral calculi.

Mesenteric Arteriogram

- For possible radiologic intervention after positive tagged GI bleeding study.

- Interventional radiology will rarely perform an arteriogram for GI bleeding without a recent tagged RBC scan.

- Sensitivity is 1 cc/min (tagged RBC scan is more sensitive).

24

Interventional Radiology

Joseph V. Philip

Before calling the interventional radiologist, you must know the following information:

- Platelet count
- INR and PTT
- Serum creatinine
- Allergy to IV dye?
- Allergy to antibiotics (usually given before abscess drainage, biliary procedures, GI procedures, and genitourinary procedures)?
- Current anticoagulation therapy (heparin, warfarin, antiplatelet agents) (Table 24-1)
- Presence of inferior vena cava filter
- NPO status (required for conscious sedation)
- Current bacteremia (permanent and long-term implantable devices are contraindicated in bacteremic patients)
- Who will give consent?

VENOUS ACCESS

The interventional radiology service will want to know what the line will be used for, for how long, and how many lumens are required.

- Nontunneled lines can be used for days to a few months. The double-lumen Hohn is a general-purpose, nontunneled catheter. Other non-tunneled catheters include Hemocath (for pheresis) and Quinton (hemodialysis).
- Tunneled catheters are for longer-term placement. They include Hickman (usually dual lumen; triple lumen available), Neostar (triple-lumen pheresis), Ash (hemodialysis), and Groshong (hemodialysis).
- PICC (peripherally inserted central catheter) lines are an option for a few days to a couple of weeks, but they often fail if needed for longer.

TABLE 24-1.
INTERVENTIONAL RADIOLOGY PARAMETERS
AT THE MALLINCKRODT INSTITUTE OF RADIOLOGY
AT BARNES-JEWISH HOSPITAL, ST. LOUIS

Vascular access		
Arterial		
Elective	INR <2.25	Platelets >80,000
	Heparin turned off 4 hrs prior	
Emergent	INR <2.75	Platelets >50,000
If	INR >2.75	Platelets <50,000
then	Leave sheath in place and observe patient in ICU	
Venous	INR <4.25	Platelets >50,000
	Heparin turned off when patient called for procedure	
Nontunneled central lines	INR <4.25	Platelets >25,000
Tunneled central lines	INR <2.25	Platelets >50,000
Nonvascular procedure	INR <1.75	Platelets >80,000
	Heparin turned off 4 hrs prior	

PULMONARY ANGIOGRAPHY

Let the interventionalist know:

- Whether an inferior vena cava filter is desired if the angiogram is positive for pulmonary embolism.

- If pulmonary arterial pressure measurements are needed.

- If left bundle branch block is present (raises risk of complete heart block when the wires and catheter are passed through the right heart).

ABSCESS DRAINAGE

Although the particular catheter type, number, size, and number of side holes vary according to the clinical situation, the general approach to fluid collection drainage is the same. The main limitation is safe approach to the fluid collection.

- The fluid collection is localized by ultrasound, fluoroscopy, and/or CT. The fluid collection may be aspirated for gross evaluation before deciding on placement of a drainage catheter. The drainage catheter is placed over a guidewire (Seldinger technique).

- When drain output reduces or stops, the cause must be considered. Possibilities include the catheter tip's migrating outside of the fluid collection, catheter blockage, or resolution of the collection. Persistent fluid drainage raises the possibility of an enteric fistula. Fluoroscopic catheter injection or CT may be used to investigate.

- Catheters can be removed when the patient has improved clinically and drain output is negligible. Removal should be done in consultation with the interventional team that placed the catheter. An imaging study is often performed to document resolution of the collection before catheter removal.

25

Vascular Studies

Nirmal K. Veeramachaneni

. . . red means away from the heart, blue means toward the heart . . .

The most common problems of the vascular system are atherosclerosis with resulting peripheral vascular disease, thromboembolic disease, venous insufficiency, and venous occlusion. Tests to evaluate **arterial** problems include the following.

ANGIOGRAPHY

Angiography is the gold standard in the evaluation of arteriooocclusive disease. It provides accurate visualization of the degree of insult to the arterial lumen and a road map for eventual revascularization. Not all patients require angiography.

SEGMENTAL SYSTOLIC PRESSURES/ ANKLE BRACHIAL INDEX

Segmental systolic pressures/ankle brachial index (ABI) are simple and effective methods to determine the degree of vascular occlusion. Arterial pressures are determined in the arms, proximal and distal thighs, and proximal and distal calves. Comparing pressures between the same points on two extremities, or between two successive points on an extremity, helps define the location of obstruction. Values are normalized by dividing the ankle pressure by the brachial pressure. This study may be done at the bedside using a Doppler probe; when the dorsalis pedis/ posterior tibial pulse is regained on deflation of the BP cuff placed on the ankle, that is the systolic pressure at the ankle. This study is often coupled with a standard exercise regimen. Normal limbs without arterial obstruction have unchanged pressures after exertion, whereas obstruction leads to a dramatic drop in the ABI. The reflexive vasodilation of hypoxic tissues is responsible for this phenomenon. In general, symptoms of claudication arise in those with an ABI <0.7, and rest pain in those with ABI <0.4. An ABI >0.9 is considered normal. Those with calcified vessels, such as diabetics, frequently have ABIs >1.

PLETHYSMOGRAPHY

Plethysmography is a method of determining the volume of blood that passes a given point. The method relies on measuring the pressure exerted by the arterial pulse on an inflated cuff as a measure of volume change. The usual peripheral vascular pattern is a dicrotic notch, a rapid upslope with a sharp peak, and a downslope with a notch representing flow reversal in early diastole. This is also evident on Doppler examination: The audible triphasic pulsation consists of rapid acceleration, a short period of reversal, and a return in forward flow throughout the remainder of diastole. Obstruction leads to loss of the triphasic signal, with a resulting dampened monophasic or complete loss of signal.

DUPLEX ULTRASOUND

Duplex ultrasound combines ultrasound imaging with Doppler flow detection. In well-trained hands, it is an accurate method of detecting and imaging areas of stenosis. It is most commonly used to evaluate the carotid artery, and many centers use it as the sole preoperative evaluation of carotid disease.

Tests to evaluate **venous** problems include the following.

VENOGRAMS

Venograms remain the gold standard for evaluating the venous system; however, they are rarely performed, except in the evaluation of vascular access for hemodialysis (fistulogram). Dialysis access dysfunction may be the result of inflow problems with stenosis at the arterial end or outflow problems with stenosis, aberrant collateral flow, or thrombosis of the venous limb.

DUPLEX ULTRASOUND

Duplex ultrasound of the venous system has become the standard for evaluation of deep vein thrombosis. Detection of venous thrombosis below the knee is less reliable than above the knee. Ultrasound cannot be used to evaluate the pelvic veins.

IMPEDANCE PLETHYSMOGRAPHY

Impedance plethysmography is rarely performed because of the increased accuracy of other methods for evaluation of deep vein thrombosis. It operates on the principle that clotting causes engorgement of the vein and extremity. An extremity's change in volume with application and rapid release of a tourniquet is measured.

V

Common Calls

. . . house officer notified; no new orders . . .

26 Common Calls: General Procedure

Emily R. Winslow

Calls from the nurse on a busy call night, especially about patients with whom you are not familiar, are a constant source of frustration. However, even the most trivial of calls can lead to important discoveries that may significantly change a patient's management. The most important point is to **go see the patient.** If the problem is not acute, you may be able to delay until you finish whatever more pressing matter you are dealing with, but don't forget to see the patient as soon as possible.

The usual scenario is that a nurse will call with an abnormal finding or complaint. Do not be fooled into thinking that the nurse knows the diagnosis; he or she is only giving you the data. Although you must address the symptom, your primary objective is to uncover the underlying problem. In other words, you must make the diagnosis.

How you respond to each of these calls depends on a variety of factors and most certainly will evolve over the course of your training. Initially, you will need to let your senior resident know about any significant patient changes. Gradually, you will be allowed more responsibility and will be better equipped to handle common problems. In addition, how well you know the patient will influence how you investigate the problem.

The format we suggest has been used for the more complex problems. We begin each with a set of bullet points: *key thoughts, tests, and interventions* with which to begin. Once the patient has been stabilized, you can take the time to read the rest of that section.

We chose this format to conveniently present the information in an orderly, reproducible fashion. Many problems should not be approached in this order. For example, a chart review should not be the first step in the care of an unstable patient.

- **Approach each patient with common sense as your guide. Never delay personally evaluating a sick patient. When in doubt, go to the bedside first.**

- **Most testing (exclusive of lab work and plain x-rays) and interventions should be discussed with a senior resident before being performed.**

INITIAL CALL

- When the nurse calls, you need to get the necessary information to be able to prioritize the problem. The most important information is the patient's current vital signs and the chief complaint.

- The nurse's sense of urgency about the problem may help you sort out how soon you need to see the patient. If the call warrants an immediate trip to the bedside, go to the patient's room directly.

- Ask the nurse to get the chart and whatever other equipment you will need (e.g., ECG machine, IV fluids) and meet you at the bedside.

- Do not worry about getting a detailed medical history or other information until the life-threatening problem is settled.

CHART REVIEW

If the problem is not life threatening, your time is best spent by going to the chart and gathering basic information about the patient. This should include the following:

- Operation and postoperative day.

- Indication for operation.

- Postoperative course and any complications.

- Significant medical history.

- Current medications, diet orders, and lab results.

HISTORY

- When going into the room, introduce yourself to the patient and explain that you have been called because the nurse is concerned about whatever issue you are there to settle.

- Then give the patient time to tell you what is wrong. The patient usually can provide you with the most important information.

- Make sure to take a focused history relevant to the problem you are investigating.

PHYSICAL EXAM

- *Always* examine the patient.

- Do so in adequate light, even if it is very late at night and the patient's roommate is sleeping.

- Make sure to look at the operative site. Take the dressing down if you need to.

- Always look at the drains and the fluid in them.

DIFFERENTIAL DIAGNOSIS

After you have the basic information, you should be able to generate a differential diagnosis. Think carefully; this is the critical step in evaluating all patient problems. If you don't consider a particular diagnosis, you are likely to miss it.

TESTING

You should next decide what ancillary testing is needed. If the patient needs a chest x-ray, don't be afraid to tell the nurse that it needs to be done right away. Don't wait until morning because it may inconvenience the staff or the patient.

TREATMENT

Some benign problems require nothing more than reassurance. However, serious problems commonly occur on a surgical service, and your treatment plan may save a patient's life. Possible treatments include medications, bedside procedures, and reoperation. In addition, the patient may require transfer to a more closely monitored setting, such as an ICU.

What follow in the next chapters are the most common problems experienced on a surgical service. Ultimately, you will develop your own method of dealing with each. Here, we present efficient and effective management summaries for these common issues.

27

Chest Pain

Emily R. Winslow

- **Hemodynamic instability?**
- **ECG**
- **Oxygen**
- **Nitroglycerin**
- **Troponin-I and/or CK-MB**
- **CBC**
- **Chest x-ray**
- **IV access**

The usual response to a call from a nurse concerning a patient with chest pain is to ask for vital signs and a stat ECG. Go directly to the patient's room. Have someone bring you the chart.

CHART REVIEW

- History of coronary artery disease and previous interventions (cardiac catheterizations, coronary artery bypass grafting).
- Home cardiac medications.
- Inpatient cardiac medications.
- Recent cardiac stresses (e.g., tachycardia, prolonged OR time).

HISTORY

- **Nature of pain:** Pressure, crushing, tearing, burning.
- **Location of pain:** Substernal, jaw, left arm.
- **Duration of pain:** How long has the pain been there?
- **Similar pains in past:** Has the patient felt anything similar in the past?

- **Difficulty breathing:** Is the patient short of breath? Is there a pleuritic component to the chest pain?

- **Exacerbating factors:** Does anything seem to make the pain worse, such as movement of the arm, sitting up, or walking to the bathroom?

PHYSICAL EXAM

- **Overall appearance:** In a patient with chest pain, the most telling feature of the physical exam is the view from the end of the bed. A pale and distressed-looking patient will alert you to a more serious problem that needs immediate intervention.

- **Pulmonary:** Listen for rales, wheezes, basilar crackles, or rubs.

- **Cardiac:** Listen for the heart rate, rhythm, and new murmurs.

- **Recent procedures:** Look for signs of recent line placement or attempts and such procedures as thoracentesis and chest tube insertion or removal.

DIFFERENTIAL DIAGNOSIS

- **Cardiac ischemia:** Patients who have undergone a major operation have been placed under significant physiologic stress. It is not uncommon for patients with angina to have an exacerbation of their condition in the postoperative period. Such an exacerbation will usually be fairly obvious, in that this group will describe the pain as similar to their previous angina, and it will usually be relieved by nitroglycerin.

- **Myocardial infarction (MI):** There is a critical difference between the patient with angina and the patient who has had or is having an MI. MI patients will have pain that is more severe than their typical anginal pain, and the symptoms will last longer. In addition, they will usually not respond completely to nitroglycerin. However, the key feature in distinguishing the angina patient from the MI patient is the difference in the ECG. Most major MIs will change the ECG ST wave segments in the territory of the vessel that is occluded.

- **Pneumothorax (PTX):** The patient may have a noncardiac cause of chest pain. Patients who have had recent procedures (central lines, thoracentesis, chest tube removals) or even failed attempts at these procedures are at risk of developing a PTX. In addition, any patient with intrinsic lung disease who has been intubated and undergone positive pressure ventilation in the OR may develop a PTX. You will be able to recognize it by listening to the patient's chest closely and by examining the chest x-ray.

- **Pulmonary embolism (PE):** Surgical patients are at increased risk of deep venous thrombosis and therefore of PE. These patients may describe chest pain, rather than shortness of breath, as their most prominent symptom. Always have a low threshold for considering PE in a patient with chest pain that is pleuritic in nature.

- **Aortic dissection:** Aortic dissection is much more uncommon, but you may encounter it in blunt trauma patients. Usually, it is described as an intrascapular ripping or tearing pain. It is a true emergency, so any suspicion of aortic dissection warrants an immediate call to a more senior resident.

- **Gastroesophageal reflux:** Patients who have undergone intra-abdominal surgery will often have some symptoms of reflux during their postoperative course. It will present as a burning or warm feeling in the lower chest. Any patient who has had antireflux surgery (e.g., Nissen or Toupet fundoplication) and complains of chest pain should be suspected of having a slipped wrap (intrathoracic migration) or esophageal perforation until proven otherwise. It requires an upper GI contrast study and/or CT scan.

- **Rib fractures:** In the multitrauma patient and patients who have undergone CPR, the presence of rib fractures is often overlooked in the search for life-threatening injuries. However, they will cause the patient great discomfort and are diagnosed by chest x-ray and/or rib films.

TESTING

- **Labs:** Cardiac enzymes (troponin-I, CK-MB), CBC, and electrolytes.

- **ECG:** All patients need an immediate ECG that should be compared to any available old ECG.

- **Chest x-ray:** Patients suspected of having a PTX or a PE should have a stat portable chest x-ray. Do not send patients with chest pain off the floor.

- **Rib films:** Get in patients with suspected rib fractures.

- **V̇/Q̇ scan or PE-protocol CT:** Order in patients suspected of having a PE. Check with a senior resident first.

TREATMENT

- **Oxygen**

- **Nitroglycerin:** Sublingual nitroglycerin should be your first-line therapy for patients suspected of having cardiac-related chest pain. Give 0.4 mg sublingually q5mins × three doses. Be cautious of the patient with aortic stenosis.

- **Morphine:** IV morphine is essential in the treatment of cardiac-related chest pain. Remember to use it cautiously in the elderly patient with narcotics already on board (e.g., a patient with patient-controlled analgesia) and in patients with renal failure.

- **Aspirin:** A patient with chest pain that is cardiac in etiology should receive two chewable aspirin (81 mg each) as soon as possible. Many postoperative patients can tolerate this mild anticoagulation, but in patients with a high risk of bleeding, check with your senior resident first.

- **Antacids:** Patients suspected of having simple reflux-related chest pain can be treated acutely with liquid antacids and should be placed on H_2-blockers.

- **Chest tube placement:** A chest tube is necessary for any patient with a large and/or symptomatic PTX.

- **Anticoagulation:** If a PE is highly suspected, consider immediate anticoagulation. This is always a difficult decision in the postoperative patient who is at risk for bleeding and should never be done without first consulting a senior resident.

- **Cardiology consultation:** If a patient is showing signs of an MI or has coronary artery disease with angina at rest, you will need the help of a cardiologist. Remember that any patient suspected of having cardiac chest pain must be made chest pain free. If this cannot be accomplished rapidly (within 20–30 mins), you will likely need cardiac consultation.

28

Confusion, Mental Status Change, and Agitation

Jeremy Goodman

- **Lateralizing neurologic deficits**
- **Vital signs**
- **Oxygen saturation**
- **Fingerstick glucose**
- **CBC**
- **Chemistry panel**

General anesthesia, narcotics, loss of a normal orienting environment, and disruption of the normal sleep-wake cycle contribute to the frightening loss of mental faculties. Nothing is scarier for a patient than to be in a strange place, in pain, and completely disoriented. Don't forget the family, either, who is seeing a loved one change before their eyes.

Understand that the confused patient will always be frightened and sometimes verbally and physically abusive. Try to get a sense of whether the patient's disorientation includes paranoia, which will make the situation more difficult. It may be difficult to get direct answers from these patients, but try to gain an idea of the severity of their mental deficit.

CHART REVIEW

- Type and quantity of anesthetic drugs and postoperative narcotics and sedatives.

- History of neurologic disorders, such as senile dementia, Alzheimer's disease, or seizures.

- History of alcohol use.

- History of prescription or illicit psychoactive drug use.

HISTORY

- Ask the typical "alert and oriented ×3" questions: name, place, and date.

- Does the patient understand the reason for being in the hospital?

- Find out from the nurses or family members if the patient fell or if there was some other precipitating event.

PHYSICAL EXAM

- Look for signs of lateralizing neurologic findings. A facial droop, slurred speech, or weak extremity strongly suggests a stroke.

- Examine incisions and catheter sites for evidence of infection.

- Examine the head for evidence of a fall that has led to intracranial injury.

DIFFERENTIAL DIAGNOSIS

- **Hypoxemia:** Low oxygen saturation can lead to mental status changes, so remember to determine and correct the underlying cause of hypoxemia.

- **Hypoglycemia**

- **Stroke or transient ischemic attack:** Suggested by lateralizing neurologic signs, as mentioned under Physical Exam.

- **Seizure:** The classic seizure pattern includes a postictal stage of variable length characterized by lethargy and confusion.

- **Infection:** Mental status changes may be the only indication of occult infection.

- **Medication:** Especially narcotics and anesthetic agents.

- **Alcohol or substance withdrawal**

- **"ICU psychosis" or "sundowning":** More often found in elderly patients who have been in the ICU or otherwise loud and disorienting settings. It is a diagnosis of exclusion.

TESTING

- **Pulse oximetry:** Hypoxemia is a dangerous cause of confusion.

- **Bedside glucose check:** Should be performed immediately, as hypoglycemia is an easily correctable cause of confusion.

- **Electrolytes:** Order a chemistry panel to check for hypo- or hypernatremia or hypercalcemia.

- **CBC:** An elevated WBC count will help lead to the diagnosis of infection. Blood cultures can also be obtained.

- **Drug levels:** If the patient takes anticonvulsants, check serum levels of those drugs.

- **Head CT:** Have a low threshold for requesting a noncontrast head CT to rule out bleeding or elevated intracranial pressure. Check with a senior resident first.

- **Lumbar puncture:** Although the incidence of meningitis or sub-arachnoid hemorrhage is quite low on a surgical service, a lumbar puncture is at times indicated. Check with a senior resident first.

TREATMENT

- **Ensure the patient's safety:** Sometimes a soothing voice or the presence of a family member is all it takes to calm the agitated patient. If necessary, physical and/or chemical restraints can be used temporarily, but only as a last resort. Restraining a patient is a serious matter and should be accompanied by frequent reevaluations.

- **Administer supplemental oxygen and dextrose as indicated.** Correction of electrolytes should also be undertaken. Once the patient recovers, do not forget to assess for the underlying cause of the metabolic disturbance.

- **Acute stroke:** Acute stroke is an indication for an emergency neurology consult. A minority of patients may be candidates for thrombolytic therapy and anticoagulation. Once the diagnosis of stroke is confirmed, request physical, occupational, and/or speech therapy consults.

- **Alcohol withdrawal:** Alcohol withdrawal can lead to life-threatening delirium tremens if not recognized and treated promptly. Benzodiazepines are used for agitation, and clonidine (Catapres) may be added to prevent or treat sympathetic hyperactivity.

- **Treat infections as indicated.** Indwelling central lines should be changed, and empiric antibiotics may be started if suspicion is high. Remember to obtain microbiology studies before the first dose of antibiotic is administered.

- **Get a sitter.** If the patient remains a threat to self or others, consider asking a staff member to stay in the room. This "sitter" can verbally redirect the patient and prevent him or her from pulling out tubes and lines.

- **Medications should be used cautiously and sparingly for agitation.** Check with a senior resident first.

  - Benzodiazepines: Very effective when administered IV. Should be avoided in the elderly.

- Haloperidol (Haldol): This antipsychotic can be given IV, or IM if the patient has pulled out the IV. Should be avoided in the elderly. May cause cardiac arrhythmias.

- Atypical antipsychotics: PO drugs such as olanzapine (Zyprexa), risperidone (Risperdal), and quetiapine (Seroquel) are generally safer in the elderly but require several days to take effect.

- **Minimize disruptions and maintain a normal sleep-wake cycle.** If the patient is hemodynamically stable, you may be able to decrease the frequency of vital sign measurements. Move the patient closer to a window, minimize noise, and keep the lights off overnight.

29

Constipation

Nirmal K. Veeramachaneni

- **Rule out obstruction before giving laxatives**
- **Rectal exam**

Just as diarrhea is bothersome to the patient, lack of a bowel movement may be just as unpleasant. As with diarrhea, it is important to define what constipation means. The usual definition is <2 bowel movements/ wk. The symptoms often expressed include a sensation of bloating, need to strain, and hard or pellet-like stools. What is perceived as constipation by one patient is normal for another.

CHART REVIEW

- History of GI surgery.
- History of bowel disorders, such as inflammatory bowel disease or irritable bowel syndrome.
- Home medication list, focusing on laxatives.
- Current medication list, focusing on narcotics and other constipating agents.

HISTORY

- When was the last normal bowel movement?
- What are the patient's normal bowel habits?
- Does the patient use prescription or over-the-counter laxatives at home?

PHYSICAL EXAM

- **Abdominal exam, including rectal exam:** Look for masses, fecal impaction, and perianal pathology.

DIFFERENTIAL DIAGNOSIS

- **Medications:** Opiates, tricyclic antidepressants, antipsychotics, and muscle relaxants.

- **Mechanical:** Bowel obstruction or fecal impaction. Remember that ostomies can become blocked by undigested food or stool.

- **Oncologic:** Mass lesions with luminal blockage or extrinsic compression.

- **Neurogenic disorders:** Autonomic neuropathy, diabetes, and spinal cord disorders.

- **Endocrine:** Hypercalcemia and hypothyroidism.

- **Perianal disease:** Pain from fissures, abscesses, or hemorrhoids can cause reluctance to defecate, eventually leading to constipation.

TESTING

- **Lab studies:** The clinical setting should determine the need for lab evaluation, as blood work is rarely necessary for constipation.

- **X-ray:** Radiographic evaluation, such as an obstructive series, is useful if you are concerned about more pathologic causes, such as bowel obstruction, abscess, or perforation. An abdominal x-ray will also reveal a stool-filled colon. Contrast enema studies may be both diagnostic and therapeutic.

- **Colonoscopy:** More useful in the setting of chronic constipation. Invasive and protracted studies, such as colonoscopy, anal manometry, and transit time, may be necessary in the outpatient setting. Check with a senior resident before ordering.

TREATMENT

- **Manual disimpaction:** For fecal impaction, this involves removing the stool from the rectal vault with your fingers.

- **Bulk-forming laxatives:**

  - Psyllium (Metamucil), methylcellulose (Citrucel).

  - Generally safe, but the patient must drink fluids or the symptoms will worsen.

  - Should not be given in the recent postoperative period.

- **Hyperosmolar/emollient laxatives:**

  - Lactulose, sorbitol, mineral oil.

  - These agents are poorly absorbed and partially metabolized by bacteria, leading to bloating and flatulence.

  - Mineral oil has the potential of causing lipoid pneumonitis if aspirated.

  - Should not be given in the recent postoperative period.

- **Docusate (Colace):** Used to soften stool, presumably by reducing surface tension and permitting the penetration of the fecal mass by intestinal fluid. Its value is uncertain.

- **Magnesium citrate:** Saline-based osmotic laxative that may lead to electrolyte imbalance, such as hypermagnesemia, in patients with renal failure.

- **Polyethylene glycol solution (GoLYTELY):** An isoosmotic solution that induces diarrhea without change in fluid/ion balance. It is most often used as a bowel prep. Large volumes are required (4 L) and should not be used in patients with gastric retention.

- **Enemas:** These are safe to administer in most patients.

  - Tap water enemas may cause dilutional hyponatremia and neurologic symptoms.

  - Phosphate-based enemas (Fleet's) may cause hypocalcemia and hyperphosphatemia, especially in patients with renal dysfunction.

  - Should not be given in the recent postoperative period.

- **Stimulants**

  - Bisacodyl (Dulcolax), cascara, senna, castor oil.

  - Act by irritating colonic mucosa. Side effects include pain and cramping.

30

Diarrhea

Nirmal K. Veeramachaneni

- **Fluid status**
- **Electrolytes**
- ***Clostridium difficile***

Just as all that wheezes is not asthma, all that flows is not diarrhea. By definition, diarrhea is either an abnormal number of bowel movements (>3/day) or quantity of stool (>200 g/day). There is incredible patient variation. Some will complain of diarrhea and mean a single loose bowel movement. For the purposes of this discussion, we define the complaint of diarrhea to include abnormally elevated enteric output (per rectum or ostomy).

CHART REVIEW

- Is there a history of GI surgery?
- Is there a history of bowel disorders, such as inflammatory bowel disease or irritable bowel syndrome?
- Has there been recent antibiotic use?

HISTORY

- How long has the diarrhea been going on?
- How many stools/day?
- What is the character of the stool?
- Has there been any blood per rectum?

PHYSICAL EXAM

- Assess volume status by exam of mucous membranes and skin turgor.
- A rectal/stomal exam is important, as it is possible to identify occult tumors, or even partially obstructing fecaliths causing frequent, watery stools. *Use caution*: In the immediate postoperative period,

it is possible to put your finger through an anastomotic line! Check with your senior resident before performing a rectal exam in the postoperative period in a patient with a low rectal anastomosis.

DIFFERENTIAL DIAGNOSIS

- **Infection:** Most commonly *Clostridium difficile* colitis in the hospitalized surgical patient.

- **Ileostomy and postcolectomy states:** Loss of the colon leads to approximately 1.5 L of small intestinal succus with no means of controlled expulsion. Normal bowel habits with an ileostomy are approximately 1 L of stoma output/day. Loss of the rectum usually leads to 6–7 bowel movements/day.

- **Medications:** Many drugs can cause GI upset and diarrhea. Antibiotics may directly cause diarrhea or predispose to the development of *C. difficile* colitis.

- **Dumping syndrome:** A range of symptoms occurs in all individuals after gastric surgery. They include epigastric fullness, nausea, vomiting, crampy abdominal pain, bloating, and diarrhea. These are often accompanied by vasomotor symptoms. The classic history is the presentation of symptoms shortly after eating.

- **Pancreatic insufficiency:** Leads to malabsorption and steatorrhea (fatty stool).

- **Ischemic states:** Intestinal angina may be the result of vessel occlusion. This is especially true after aortic surgery or in patients with atrial fibrillation. Pain usually accompanies it.

- **Diet sensitivity:** Lactose intolerance or gluten sensitivity.

- **Obstruction:** Intestinal obstruction can eventually lead to diarrhea as backed-up fluid overflows the blockage.

TESTING

- ***C. difficile* toxin assay:** Should be sent for any surgical patient with a history of recent antibiotic use. Three consecutive daily samples yield the highest sensitivity.

- **Electrolytes:** Diarrhea is bicarbonate and potassium rich and can lead to electrolyte disturbances. Significant fluid loss can also induce prerenal azotemia.

TREATMENT

1. **Maintain hydration:** Supplemental IV fluid may be necessary if the patient is not able to keep up with fluid losses. Consider replacement of actual measured losses.

2. **Electrolyte replacement:** As indicated based on the electrolyte panel.

3. **Antibiotics:** Eliminate antibiotics if possible. A strong suspicion or confirmed diagnosis of *C. difficile* colitis should prompt the administration of PO metronidazole (Flagyl). IV metronidazole may be given if the PO route is not available. PO vancomycin (Vancocin) is a second-line agent.

4. **Constipating agents:** Fiber, atropine/diphenoxylate (Lomotil), loperamide (Imodium), or opiates may be given to the patient with noninfectious diarrhea. These drugs should not be used in *C. difficile* colitis, as they may cause enterotoxin to accumulate. Check with your senior resident.

5. **Evaluate diet:** Confirm that your patient does not have sensitivity to the foods he or she is being given. Postgastrectomy patients may benefit from multiple small meals throughout the day instead of the standard three meals a day.

6. **Colonoscopy/proctoscopy:** More invasive studies such as these are appropriate in the proper setting (e.g., investigation for ischemia-induced diarrhea after aortic surgery). Always discuss the possibility of operative complication–induced diarrhea with your senior resident.

31

Fever

Emily R. Winslow

- **Hemodynamic instability?**
- **Postoperative day**
- **Operative site/wound appearance**
- **CBC**
- **Antibiotics**

Although the request for an acetaminophen order may seem mundane, you can make a real difference in the care of a postoperative patient with a fever. Getting therapy started early for infectious problems is essential. We generally consider a significant fever to be ≥101.5°F (38.6°C).

CHART REVIEW

- Essential to note: preexisting pulmonary disease, immunocompromised state (diabetes, steroids, immunosuppressants, postsplenectomy), and allergies to antibiotics.

- Go through the daily notes to see if the patient has had other fevers and what workup has already been done (UA, sputum cultures, chest x-ray, blood cultures, CT scan). Check to see if the patient is currently on antimicrobial therapy.

HISTORY

- **Mental status:** Confusion is one of the first signs of a serious infection (ask basic questions of orientation).

- **Pulmonary complaints:** Ask about cough, sputum production, and shortness of breath. Ask the patient to use the incentive spirometer and assess whether the patient can take in an adequate tidal volume.

- **Abdominal pain:** May be very subjective. However, if you sense that the patient is having increasing discomfort or is not following the typical course for his or her operation, be concerned about the possibility of an intraabdominal infection.

- **GI complaints:** Ask about nausea and vomiting. Always ask specifically about diarrhea and its color and consistency.

- **Urinary complaints:** If the patient does not have a Foley catheter, ask about such UTI symptoms as urgency, burning, or frequency. In a man, you should ask if he has symptoms of prostate enlargement (weak stream, incomplete emptying, frequent urination).

- **Lower extremity complaints:** Ask about the sense of swelling or pain in either leg, particularly the calves.

PHYSICAL EXAM

- **Indwelling foreign object:** Determine how long the line or catheter has been in place.

  - Central lines, IVs, epidural catheters: Look at the site carefully.

  - Foley catheter: Character of the urine.

  - Abdominal drains: Character of the fluid.

- **Pulmonary exam:** Auscultate the chest for findings that suggest a developing pneumonia or generalized crackles to suggest atelectasis. Measure the oxygen saturation.

- **Abdominal exam:** Rule out peritoneal irritation and inflammation. Watch for localized tenderness in the right upper quadrant to suggest cholecystitis or suprapubic tenderness to suggest a UTI.

- **Wound:** Look closely at the patient's wound. *Take down the dressing.* If it is within the first 48 hrs, you should do so with sterile gloves on and then replace it with a sterile dressing. Look for erythema or discharge. If the wound is packed, change the packing and assess the quality of the fluid in the wound. Always think about the possibility of wound dehiscence and evisceration.

- **Lower extremities:** Look for swelling, tenderness, or erythema to suggest a deep vein thrombosis.

DIFFERENTIAL DIAGNOSIS

- **Atelectasis:** Atelectasis is the collapse of terminal airways that often occurs in surgical patients. The predisposing factors include lying supine, being unable to take deep breaths or sigh (usually secondary to incisional pain), and a prolonged period of time on the operating table. Atelectasis alone does not cause extreme temperature elevations, and it will *never* make the patient look sick or have other abnormal vital signs. You should never feel satisfied with the diagnosis of atelectasis; it is a diagnosis of exclusion when the rest of your search uncovers nothing. Atelectasis is most commonly seen on postoperative day 1.

- **Urinary infection:** Patients with indwelling catheters have a high risk of bacterial seeding and subsequent UTI. In men, urinary retention from prostate enlargement is a predisposing factor to infection. If the patient has any urinary complaints or has a Foley catheter, consider a UTI. It can manifest on any postoperative day.

- **Wound infection:** Patients may develop erythema or discharge from an abdominal wound. Some very aggressive wound infections occur early in the postoperative course (e.g., *Clostridia* and *Streptococcus*). If you detect a significant amount of erythema, warmth, or any subcutaneous air on the first or second postoperative days, let your senior resident know immediately. Later, less-aggressive postoperative infections may occur. For more information on surgical site infections, see Chap. 45, Wound Drainage.

- **Pneumonia:** Suspect a pulmonary infection in patients with smoking histories, COPD, and abnormal breath sounds on physical exam. A spectrum of infection ranges from mild bronchitis to lobar consolidated pneumonia. These types of infections can occur at any time and are often dependent on preoperative pulmonary status.

- **Line infection:** If the patient has an indwelling central venous line, be concerned about the possibility of a line infection. Even if the site appears clean, the catheter tip can harbor infection. Be particularly vigilant about line infections in patients whose lines have been in for >3 days or were not placed under optimal conditions (e.g., in the ER or in the OR emergently).

- **Intraabdominal abscess:** After an abdominal operation, an intraabdominal infection might develop. It will rarely be detectable as an abscess before 5–7 days, as it takes time for a walled-off fluid collection to form. Suspect this problem in patients who had contaminated peritoneal cavities, have spiking fever patterns and rigors, and feel generally unwell.

- ***C. difficile* colitis:** *C. difficile* is a common infection in surgical patients, owing to the prevalence of antibiotic therapy. Any patient with diarrhea should be considered a possible candidate for *C. difficile* colitis. It often is associated with abdominal pain and leukocytosis.

- **Deep venous thrombosis:** Deep venous thrombosis is a common surgical problem and can cause low-grade fevers. It will not make the patient appear sick and is not likely to cause a high fever. Superficial thrombophlebitis can also cause fever, though.

- **Bacteremia/sepsis:** Any type of infection may progress to a bloodstream infection and begin to cause a systemic inflammatory response. These patients are generally sicker and have abnormal vital signs. It is essential that you recognize when a patient is beginning to become systemically ill, as these patients need to be more closely monitored and started immediately on broad-spectrum anti-biotic therapy.

- **Other:** More rare causes, but things to consider in special circum-stances, include drug reaction, Addisonian crisis, thyroid storm, pheochromocytoma, and malignant hyperthermia.

TESTING

- **CBC:** The WBC count (particularly the trend) is useful.

- **Blood cultures:** You rarely need blood cultures, but draw them if you suspect bacteremia or if the patient has an indwelling central line.

- **Urinalysis and urine culture:** Obtain from any patient with a Foley catheter or with urinary complaints.

- **Sputum culture:** Only obtain if the patient has a significant amount of sputum and is likely to have a pulmonary infection (e.g., has abnormal chest x-ray findings).

- **Chest x-ray:** Obtain on any patient with physical findings sugges-tive of pulmonary infection, shortness of breath, or hypoxemia.

- *C. difficile* **toxin assay:** Obtain on any patient with diarrhea.

- **Abdominal/pelvic CT scan:** Deciding to get a CT usually is done in consultation with a more senior resident, but think about it in patients in whom you suspect an abscess has developed.

- **Venous duplex:** Venous duplex is used to rule out a deep venous thrombosis. It can usually wait until the following morning.

TREATMENT

- If you suspect sepsis, start broad-spectrum antibiotics and consider moving the patient to a more closely monitored setting (step-down unit or ICU).

- Always order incentive spirometry and walking regimens in patients you suspect of having atelectasis.

- If you suspect a wound infection, consider opening the wound and starting antibiotics.

- In patients with a suspected pulmonary infection, initiate antimicro-bial therapy and a mobilization routine (out of bed, incentive spirometer).

- In patients with UTIs, start antibiotics and consider removing the Foley catheter or changing it if there are no contraindications to doing so.

- In patients with indwelling lines, always consider removing the line if the patient no longer needs it. If the patient needs central access, you should remove the first line and place a new one. Consider starting IV antibiotics until you get the results of blood cultures. This is best done in consultation with your senior resident.

- In a patient with suspected *C. difficile* colitis, start treatment with PO metronidazole after the stool sample has been sent.

32

Hypotension

Jeremy Goodman

- **Crash cart location**
- **Hemodynamic instability?**
- **Signs of end-organ perfusion**
- **Oxygen**
- **ECG**
- **Troponin-I and/or CK-MB**
- **Electrolytes**
- **CBC**
- **Chest x-ray**
- **IV access**

Many people live quite comfortably with a low BP. If the "alarming" value you were called about is consistent with the patient's preoperative BP, there may not be a problem. On the other hand, the chronically hypertensive patient may be symptomatic with a "normal" BP. Always consider the patient's preoperative baseline.

CHART REVIEW

- Review the patient's pre- and postoperative vital signs and urine output trends.

- Review preoperative medications. Most BP medications are given on the morning of surgery and may have long-acting properties. Be suspicious of once-a-day and extended-release preparations. Once-daily angiotensin-converting enzyme inhibitors and angiotensin II receptor blockers may be responsible for postoperative hypotension, even if the last dose was taken ≤48 hrs previously.

- Check for medication and food allergies.

- Review the operative note for any mention of complications and the anesthesia flowsheet for evidence of intraoperative BP lability. Consider that a "stable" patient being transferred from the recovery room may be supported by a lingering dose of vasopressors, which invariably wear off on arrival to the ward.

HISTORY

- Is the hypotension symptomatic (dizziness, lightheadedness, headache, sweating, or nausea)?

- Is there associated chest pain or shortness of breath?

PHYSICAL EXAM

- Look for pallor, cool extremities, dry mucous membranes, and other signs of dehydration or poor perfusion.

- Assess mental status.

- Look for evidence of drainage or swelling compartments that may indicate bleeding.

- Orthostatic vital signs may help you assess the severity of the hypotension.

- Ensure that the proper BP cuff size is used. An ill-fitting cuff will lead to false results.

DIFFERENTIAL DIAGNOSIS

- **Hypovolemic shock:** Hypovolemic shock may be due to inadequate fluid intake or excessive losses. In the immediate postoperative period, bleeding should be your primary concern.

- **Cardiogenic shock:** Intrinsic pump failure from myocardial infarction can lead to hypotension. Extrinsic pressure on the heart from tension pneumothorax or pericardial tamponade also affects BP.

- **Septic shock:** Serious and advanced infection, especially with associated bacteremia.

- **Neurogenic shock:** Primarily a concern in the spinal cord–injured patient who may have autonomic dysfunction.

- **Anaphylactic shock:** Allergic reactions can lead to life-threatening complications, including hypotension.

- **Endocrine:** Hypothyroidism or adrenal insufficiency can cause refractory hypotension.

- **Iatrogenic:** Many medications that we give patients, especially narcotics, may cause hypotension. Also, in treating the hypertensive patient, we may overshoot and cause hypotension.

- **Preoperative medications:** A diagnosis of exclusion and the result of previously taken long-acting antihypertensives. During the perioperative period, the patient's physiology changes and may demonstrate an exaggerated response to a previously stable medication regimen.

TESTING

- **CBC:** If there is any concern for ongoing blood loss or infection.

- **Cardiac evaluation:** ECG and troponin-I or CK-MB.

- **Chest x-ray:** Check chest x-ray for pneumothorax or free intraabdominal air.

- **CT:** If worried about intraabdominal or intrathoracic infection. Check with your senior resident first.

TREATMENT

- **Fluid bolus:** 500–1000 cc of normal saline can temporize the patient with hypovolemic hypotension. Remember that you may also have to increase the rate of the continuous IV infusion to avoid a recurrent problem. (See Chap. 63, Bleeding, for a thorough review of this subject.)

- **Vasopressors/inotropes:** The patient with hypotension related to cardiac failure should be managed in an ICU, although some hospitals will allow you to initiate IV pressors and inotropes on the regular ward while awaiting transfer. Dopamine (Intropin) or phenylephrine (Neo-Synephrine) may be started at low doses and titrated to maintain an acceptable BP during transfer. Check with a senior resident before administering vasoactive drugs.

- **Anaphylaxis therapy:** Severe anaphylactic reactions require transfer to a closely monitored setting. Initial treatment should consist of subcutaneous epinephrine; an H_1-blocker, such as diphenhydramine (Benadryl); an H_2-blocker, such as cimetidine (Tagamet); and IV corticosteroids. These patients usually require significant volume resuscitation as well.

- **Sepsis:** Septic shock should be treated in the ICU and requires antibiotics, fluid resuscitation, and, often, vasopressors.

- **Neurogenic shock:** Neurogenic hypotension patients may be asymptomatic and will often adjust to the lower BP over time. Acutely, treat these patients with IV fluids.

- **Hormone replacement:** Administer IV thyroid hormone and corticosteroids when appropriate.

- **Iatrogenic and preoperative medication–induced hypotension** are most often self-limited. The mainstay of treatment is cessation of the offending agent and careful observation. A small fluid bolus may be used to treat the transient hypotension.

33

Hypertension

Jeremy Goodman

- **Neurologic symptoms?**
- **Baseline BP**
- **Fluid status**

Unlike low BP, HTN is rarely an emergency. Of course, every rule has its exceptions, and patients with aortic dissections, cerebral bleeds, recent stroke, and vascular anastomoses, and those recovering from carotid surgery should not be allowed to sustain a markedly elevated BP.

You will be called frequently to address high BP, and you need to know which situations require intervention.

CHART REVIEW

- Review recent vital sign trends. See if the "alarming" BP is consistent with previous values.

- Home antihypertensive regimen.

- Inpatient antihypertensive regimen. See if it coincides with the patient's home regimen. The timing of drug administration is important as well. The patient may be due for a scheduled antihypertensive shortly.

HISTORY

- Ask about prehospital BP control. Does the patient's BP normally run high?

- Are there neurologic symptoms, such as headache, blurry vision, or dizziness?

- Is the patient experiencing chest pain or shortness of breath?

- Is there an excessive amount of pain that may be contributing to the elevated BP?

PHYSICAL EXAM

- Assess BP in both upper extremities and compare. A systolic difference of >10–20 mm Hg suggests a vascular disturbance, such as aortic dissection.
- Ensure that the proper-sized BP cuff is used.
- Perform a neurologic exam to assess for focal signs or asymmetry.

DIFFERENTIAL DIAGNOSIS

- **Pain:** Pain is the most common cause of postoperative HTN.
- **Cardiac:** Patients having myocardial ischemia or infarction may have associated HTN.
- **Essential HTN:** Remember that patients may miss scheduled doses of medications because of procedures, and GI absorption may be impaired after surgery. HTN in the postoperative period may merely reflect inadequate control of a chronic condition. It may be further exacerbated by fluid overload, usually by postoperative day 3 or 4.
- **Endocrinologic disturbances:** Rarely, profound hormone abnormalities may affect BP, as in hyperthyroidism or pheochromocytoma.

TESTING

- **Cardiac:** An ECG and cardiac enzymes should be ordered if there is concern for cardiac causes of HTN.
- **Ancillary testing:** Further ancillary testing for HTN is rarely indicated. Evaluation of essential HTN is usually not appropriate during a surgical admission.

TREATMENT

- **Analgesia:** Pain should be treated rapidly and is often all that is needed for BP control.
- **Diuresis:** By postoperative day 3 or 4, judicious use of diuretics may improve HTN exacerbated by volume overload. Check with a senior resident first.
- **Antihypertensives:** Patients with essential HTN are best treated by resuming their prehospital antihypertensive regimens. If the patient is due shortly for a scheduled antihypertensive, consider giving the dose early. Small doses of PO or IV antihypertensives are indicated for extremely high BP that has not yet responded to the patient's typical regimen. *Check with your senior resident before administering antihypertensives in the acute setting.* Remember that patients with long-standing HTN or those with cerebrovascular

or carotid disease may rely on a high cerebral perfusion pressure, and acutely dropping their BP may precipitate cerebral ischemia.

- Clonidine (Catapres): A commonly used fast-acting, short-lived PO antihypertensive. Acts as a central sympatholytic. The transdermal form is not useful acutely because of its relatively long time to onset.

- Hydralazine (Apresoline): IV direct vasodilator.

- Beta-blockers: Also very effective, but only give in a monitored setting because of their cardiac depressant and proarrhythmic potentials.

- Calcium-channel blockers: May be given IV in a monitored setting but are generally used PO for chronic HTN control.

Antihypertensive medications can be dangerous. Do not initiate them unless you are prepared to deal with the potential side effects. Most IV preparations should be used in a monitored setting.

As a general rule, you should not start new, long-term antihypertensives. It can be done, however, in consultation with the patient's primary care provider. Most patients can tolerate several days of mildly elevated BP during the postoperative period.

34 Low Urine Output

Nirmal K. Veeramachaneni

- **Foley catheter**
- **Fluid status over last 24 hrs**
- **Signs of end-organ perfusion**
- **Electrolytes**
- **CBC**

All patients requiring hospitalization for a surgical reason should have their urine output recorded. In other words, every time you write orders, you should include "strict ins and outs." This way, the problem of low urine output can be detected quickly, before renal function deteriorates.

The first question is, "How low is the urine output?" In general, we expect a euvolemic patient to make 0.5 cc of urine/kg/hr. This refers to the patient's lean body mass. So, for a patient who weighs 50 kg, the expected urine output is 25 cc/hr. In an 8-hr shift, then, the recorded value should be ≥200 cc.

Before you worry about your patient with low urine output, you should ascertain that the value is accurate. Often, it is not; patients without an indwelling Foley catheter are not in the habit of collecting their urine for measurement. Ask the following:

- Does the patient have a Foley?
- Is the patient incontinent?
- Did the patient void without having the amount measured?

The easiest way to sort this out, as always, is to go to the bedside. Ask if the patient recalls voiding without saving it. In addition, always ask if the patient currently feels the urge to void.

Assuming you have verified that the patient has low urine output, proceed with the following workup.

CHART REVIEW

- Look carefully through the patient's ins and outs over the last 48 hrs.

- Note whether the patient is receiving a diuretic of any kind or takes one at home.

- Look for the date of Foley catheter insertion or removal and information regarding whether it was a difficult Foley placement.

- Review the operative note to rule out a possible iatrogenic cause.

- Look up the patient's most recent labs, including BUN, Cr, K, and HCO_3.

- Look for any recent contrast studies.

- Review the medication list for nephrotoxins.

HISTORY

- Review for vomiting, diarrhea, or fluid loss (e.g., drains, nasogastric tube).

- Elicit symptoms of bladder outlet obstruction (slow stream, nocturia, dribbling) and ask if the patient normally takes medication for it.

- Always ask if the patient has the feeling of bladder fullness.

PHYSICAL EXAM

- Assess the patient's volume status carefully. Look for dry mucous membranes, low jugular venous pressure, decreased skin turgor, and lack of axillary sweat. These signs point toward volume depletion.

- Flush the Foley catheter with 30–50 cc of sterile water. See if it flows easily in and out of the bladder. Check the balloon valve.

- Look at the urine (if any is available). Dark colored may mean concentrated urine, but you can be fooled by pigments. A patient with elevated serum bilirubin or myoglobinuria will pass dark urine.

- Feel the suprapubic area to see if you can palpate or percuss the bladder.

DIFFERENTIAL DIAGNOSIS

Prenal: The major causes of a prerenal state are

- Volume depletion: the most common reason for surgical patients to have low urine output. To decide why a surgical patient is volume depleted, consider the following:

  - Postoperative day: Patients who are postoperative day 0–3 are still in the period of third-spacing fluids into the interstitial space. This generality applies only to patients who have undergone significant abdominal procedures.

  - Excessive losses: High NG tube output, high drain output, frequent diarrhea, or insensible losses.

- Inadequate intake: Patients whose IV fluids have been stopped but do not have sufficient PO intake may become intravascularly depleted.

- Bleeding: Patients who have lost a significant amount of blood intraoperatively or those who continue to bleed postoperatively demonstrate decreased urine output.

- Perceived volume depletion: The intravascular volume is adequate, but the kidneys are not able to sense it. The major causes of this problem are

  - Heart failure

  - Cirrhosis

Renal: This group of problems refers to patients with normal intravascular volume whose kidneys have an intrinsic problem making urine. The major causes of this type of problem include

- Acute tubular necrosis: Refers to the state in which the kidney tubules have been damaged and are unable to continue the process of properly filtering urine. Causes include

  - Prolonged hypotension (often intraoperative)

  - IV contrast loads (cardiac catheters, CT scans, angiograms)

  - Nephrotoxic drugs (aminoglycosides, amphotericin, chemotherapy)

  - Endogenous tubular toxins (myoglobinuria from muscle injuries)

- Acute interstitial nephritis: Most often due to medications like NSAIDs or beta-lactam antibiotics.

- Embolic disease: Most common in the vascular patient who had an intervention that could cause embolization of plaque and thrombus to the renal arteries. Causes include

  - Cardiac catheterization

  - Angiography

  - Left heart thrombi from large myocardial infarctions or atrial fibrillation

- Graft dysfunction: Patients with newly transplanted kidneys fall into their own class when they have the problem of low urine output. One of the possible etiologies is intrinsic graft dysfunction. Other things to consider are acute vascular problems, such as renal artery thrombosis and anastomotic disruption of the ureter. Do not treat these patients like others with low urine output. Alert your senior resident immediately.

Postrenal: *Postrenal* refers to patients who make adequate urine at the level of the kidney but have some problem that does not allow the urine to exit through the urethra. Multiple possible etiologies exist:

- Ureter problems: Surgically transected ureters, extrinsically compressed ureters (blood clots, retroperitoneal fibrosis), and luminally blocked ureters (stones, clots) can cause a decrease in urine output.

- Bladder problems: Usually a bladder outlet obstruction issue; easily relieved by placing a Foley catheter.

- Prostate problems: These patients usually give a history of prostate enlargement. Placement of a standard Foley may be difficult, requiring a stiffer catheter (coudé) or even a urology consult.

- Catheter problem: The catheter is blocked with debris and not properly draining urine from the bladder, or it is malpositioned.

TESTING

- **Chemistries:** BUN, Cr, K, HCO$_3$. Chemistries can help you assess the severity of renal compromise (i.e., whether the patient has developed acute renal failure) and the potential for complications (the development of hyperkalemia). Urine electrolytes (Na, Cr) can also be measured.

- **CBC:** Order a CBC when you suspect the patient may be volume depleted as a result of blood loss.

- **Urine sediment:** If you suspect a patient of having acute tubular necrosis, the best diagnostic test is urine sediment, looking for "muddy brown casts." If you suspect acute interstitial nephritis, send urine for eosinophil measurement.

- **Urine specific gravity:** Highly concentrated urine suggests intravascular depletion.

- **Renal ultrasound:** Ultrasound is almost never needed in the middle of the night but is a test to consider performing the next morning if things have not improved. It will tell you if there is hydronephrosis, which suggests a postrenal cause.

TREATMENT

- **Bolus of isotonic IV fluid:** The most frequent and successful treatment you will offer the surgical patient. A good start is 500 mL of normal saline. However, do not simply "bolus the patient" without first considering comorbidities like congestive heart failure. Don't bolus with $1/2$ normal saline or any fluid with added potassium.

- **Change the fluid balance:** If your patient is volume depleted because of increased losses, just giving a bolus may only fix the problem transiently. The best way to deal with this is to replace whatever fluid is being lost. If the patient appears to be third-spacing fluid, consider either increasing the rate of maintenance fluid or changing to an isotonic solution.

- **Insert a Foley:** Any patient with low urine output who does not respond to conservative measures should have a Foley catheter inserted for closer monitoring. In addition, a Foley catheter may definitively treat a patient with postrenal obstruction.

- **Ensure proper Foley function:** Always flush the Foley to ensure that it is patent and the catheter will return the amount of fluid you have flushed. If this does not occur, you should manipulate or change it until you are assured that the catheter is adequately draining the bladder.

- **Medications:** If the patient not only has low urine output but also appears to be experiencing a change in renal function (increasing Cr), you should discontinue any medications that could be contributing to the problem. In addition, adjust any medications that require renal dosing accordingly.

- **Diuretics:** It is often tempting to give a patient who does not respond to several boluses of fluid a dose of furosemide (Lasix) to see if the urine output will improve. This is, at times, the correct management decision, but it is not one that you should make without very careful consideration. Giving IV fluids followed by diuretics does not improve renal function; it only increases urine output. The argument for doing so is that it will be easier to manage a patient who is nonoliguric than one who is oliguric. Diuretics in a hypovolemic patient worsen renal failure. Always consider central venous pressure monitoring before giving diuretics if the patient's volume status is unclear. Always check with a more senior resident before proceeding down this path.

Nirmal K. Veeramachaneni

- **Postoperative day**
- **Type of operation**
- **Fluid status**
- **Abdominal tenderness or distention**
- **Electrolytes**

The sensation of nausea is triggered in the brain and can be due to a number of psychological and physiologic factors. The initial evaluation of the patient with nausea and vomiting (N/V) should center on differentiating the truly sick from the merely nauseated.

CHART REVIEW

- History of N/V or vertebrobasilar problems.

- History of antiemetic use.

- Allergy history: an "allergy" to narcotics often means GI upset.

HISTORY

- How long have the N/V been present?

- Are the symptoms related to food or medication intake?

- Is there a history of narcotic sensitivity?

- Has there been any hematemesis?

PHYSICAL EXAM

- **Volume status:** Look for dry mucous membranes, low jugular venous pressure, decreased skin turgor, and lack of axillary sweat. These signs point toward significant fluid loss from emesis.

- **Abdominal exam:** Assess for distention, gastric tympany, and pain.

- **Emesis:** If it has been saved, inspect the emesis for blood, color, and medication and food particles.

DIFFERENTIAL DIAGNOSIS

- **Ileus:** After any abdominal surgery, especially one in which significant dissection and manipulation have been performed, GI function will be slow to recover. Delayed gastric emptying and a bloated sensation are common and may be exacerbated by abnormal electrolytes; narcotics; antiarrhythmic agents, such as calcium-channel blockers; or infection.

- **Bowel obstruction:** This is usually accompanied by abdominal pain. Persistent emesis, prior history of obstruction, or absence of bowel movements should prompt investigation. The common causes of obstruction include adhesions, entrapment (internal or external hernias), volvulus, diverticulitis, tumors/inflammatory conditions, and abscesses.

- **Medications:** The common culprits are narcotics, anesthetics, PO potassium, and antibiotics. A temporal relationship will be evident.

- **Postoperative pain:** If severe enough, pain alone can induce N/V.

TESTING

- **Electrolytes:** With significant vomiting comes electrolyte disturbances, and a chemistry panel should be obtained.

- **CBC:** Obtain a CBC if there is any suspicion of infection.

- **Obstructive series:** To help you make the diagnosis of ileus, obstruction, or free air.

- **CT scan:** To look for intraabdominal abscess, diverticulitis, or ischemic bowel, or to further evaluate an intestinal obstruction. Check with your senior resident first.

- **Contrast enema:** For the evaluation and occasional treatment of sigmoid volvulus. Check with your senior resident first.

- **Upper GI study:** To examine esophageal and gastric motility and emptying. Check with your senior resident first.

TREATMENT

- **Nasogastric tube:** An NG tube will relieve the symptoms and can often be curative in such situations as isolated gastroparesis. In addition, the NG tube serves as a quantifiable drain, which is especially useful in guiding appropriate fluid replacement. See Part IX, Tubes and Drains, for more information.

- **Antiemetics:** A number of medications are in common use for the treatment of nausea. However, do not just order antiemetics over the phone. Examine the patient and determine whether a more serious problem exists.

- Serotonin inhibitors: Ondansetron (Zofran) and other members of its class. Very effective and very safe, but very expensive.

- Phenothiazine derivatives: These dopaminergic agents, such as prochlorperazine (Compazine) or promethazine (Phenergan), are related to a class of antipsychotics and neuroleptics. Absolute contraindications to their use include phenothiazine hypersensitivity and agranulocytosis. As their mechanism of action suggests, extrapyramidal symptoms (tardive dyskinesia and dystonia) are possible. Anticholinergic agents, such as diphenhydramine (Benadryl) or benztropine (Cogentin), can treat these acute side effects. They may also lower seizure threshold.

- Metoclopramide (Reglan): Mixed cholinergic and dopaminergic activity that serves to increase GI motility. This agent should never be used in the setting of intestinal obstruction. It has a role in diabetic gastroparesis. Extrapyramidal symptoms are also a possibility.

36

Shortness of Breath

Emily R. Winslow

- **Need for intubation**
- **Crash cart location**
- **Hemodynamic instability?**
- **Respiratory failure?**
- **Fluid status**
- **Pulse oximetry**
- **ABG**
- **ECG**
- **Chest x-ray**
- **IV access**

Your first priority is to decide whether the patient is in critical condition. This means the patient appears to be nearing respiratory failure and will need to be intubated and mechanically ventilated. If so, bypass the steps suggested below. Remember that the first two steps in the ABCs are airway and breathing.

The expression *shortness of breath* means quite different things to different patients. Sometimes, you will discover that the true complaint is chest pain, heartburn, or even a sore throat. If the patient does not appear in critical condition, proceed with the steps below.

CHART REVIEW

- History of COPD, emphysema, smoking, or congestive heart failure with pulmonary edema.

- History of deep venous thrombosis, pulmonary embolism, or inferior vena cava filter placement.

- Trend of oxygen saturations, particularly preoperatively.

- Results of most recent chest x-ray.
- Ease of intubation in OR (from anesthesia sheet).

HISTORY

- How long has the patient felt bad?
- Is the dyspnea getting better or worse?
- Has the patient ever felt this way before?
- Is there associated chest pain? Is that pain pleuritic? Palpitations?
- Have there been any recent procedures or attempts (thoracentesis, central lines)?
- Has the patient been receiving his or her home pulmonary medications, if any, while in the hospital? Have home diuretics been withheld?
- Did the onset coincide with administration of blood or a new medication?

PHYSICAL EXAM

- **Oxygen:** Make sure you know what the patient's oxygen saturation is and how much oxygen he or she is on.
- **Location of incision:** The patient who has had neck surgery represents an important subgroup with shortness of breath. In these patients, the first thing you need to do is to carefully inspect the operative site. Take the dressing down and assess whether there appears to be an underlying hematoma or mass effect. The feeling of dyspnea can result from airway compression in these patients, and its presence is a true surgical emergency. See Chap. 53, Neck, for what to do in this situation.
- **Pulmonary exam:** Listen closely for any focal findings. You need to assess whether the breath sounds are equal, whether there is dullness or hyperresonance to percussion, whether there is wheezing or stridor, and whether there are basilar rales or other abnormal lung sounds.
- **Cardiac exam:** Listen for gallops (an S_4) that can represent volume overload and congestive heart failure.
- **Lower extremities:** Look for signs of deep venous thrombosis, which can lead to pulmonary embolism.

DIFFERENTIAL DIAGNOSIS

- **Pulmonary embolism:** There are often no physical findings, so a high index of suspicion is critical. Be very concerned about patients who have hypotension or tachycardia associated with dyspnea, who complain of sudden onset shortness of breath with pleuritic chest pain, and with lower extremity signs of deep venous thrombosis. Patients at high risk for deep venous thrombosis (lower-extremity fractures, prolonged immobilization, malignancy) should also be suspected. Getting a $\dot{V}/\dot{Q}$ or CT scan is always worth considering. Remember that patients with inferior vena cava filters in place can still have a pulmonary embolism. Discuss this possibility with your senior resident immediately. Anticoagulation should not be delayed while awaiting confirmatory testing.

- **Congestive heart failure:** Surgical patients often have large fluid shifts, which can push those with decreased cardiac function into congestive heart failure. This often occurs on postoperative day 3 or 4, when the patient mobilizes fluid back into the intravascular compartment. It is also possible for a patient to be pushed into volume overload by boluses of IV fluid for low urine output or hypotension. Patients routinely on large doses of diuretics who have had them withheld postoperatively are also at risk of volume overload.

- **Exacerbation of COPD/emphysema/asthma:** Patients with underlying lung disease often have persistent or worsened symptoms while they are in the hospital. The reasons for this are multifactorial but include inadequate inhaler use, lack of routine doses of inhaled corticosteroids, and the atelectasis that most surgical patients experience.

- **Myocardial infarction:** Although most patients have associated chest pain, some present solely with shortness of breath, either as an anginal equivalent or as a result of flash pulmonary edema.

- **Pneumothorax:** Listen to breath sounds closely and determine whether there were any preceding events that could put the patient at risk (e.g., central lines, thoracentesis). Treat immediately if the patient is deteriorating.

- **Developing pneumonia:** Patients with underlying lung disease and those with prolonged illnesses may develop a hospital-acquired pneumonia. It is often associated with sputum production and focal findings on pulmonary exam. A chest x-ray is essential to making this diagnosis.

- **Arrhythmia:** Remember that a tachycardia, especially rapid atrial fibrillation, can cause shortness of breath and palpitations.

- **Neck hematoma:** See Chap. 53, Neck.

- **Anaphylaxis or allergic reaction:** Patients can develop shortness of breath as the initial expression of anaphylaxis. It is usually described as throat tightness.

TESTING

- **ABG:** Remember to record the amount of oxygen the patient is on and what the saturation reads at the time that you draw the ABG. See Appendix A, Procedures, for instructions on drawing an ABG.

- **Chest x-ray:** Mandatory in most patients with shortness of breath. Without it, you cannot exclude a pneumothorax, congestive heart failure, or pneumonia. However, even a normal x-ray will not let you off the hook; the patient with a pulmonary embolism often has a normal chest x-ray.

- **ECG:** Can help in the diagnosis of an atypical MI and of a pulmonary embolism (right-sided strain characteristics). It will also rule out rapid tachyarrhythmias. Obtain an ECG on every patient with a history of cardiac disease. Consider cardiac enzymes if the ECG is suggestive.

- **Sputum cultures:** If you think a patient has a developing pneumonia and he or she has copious sputum production, it is useful to get a sputum culture before antimicrobial treatment is initiated.

- **V̇/Q̇ scan, CT scan, or angiography:** If you suspect a pulmonary embolism, first obtain a routine chest x-ray and then proceed with the above tests. Which you obtain is situation-specific and should be discussed with a more senior resident and a radiologist.

TREATMENT

- **Oxygen:** All patients are treated with oxygen initially. Those whose oxygen saturation is persistently low after therapy should remain on it continuously.

- **Inhaled beta-agonists:** Treat any patient with wheezing or home use of inhalers with inhalers or nebulized medication early in the management of shortness of breath.

- **Morphine/nitroglycerin/diuretics:** Any patient with signs of congestive heart failure should be treated with this combination. Remember to use caution when giving surgical patients diuretics. It may be necessary to give several doses of diuretic on postoperative days 3 and 4 to avoid volume overload or to treat it once it has occurred.

- **IV heparin:** If the suspicion for a pulmonary embolus is high enough, therapy is often begun at the onset of symptoms, before diagnostic testing is performed. The postoperative patient is at risk for bleeding complications, so this must be decided carefully and with input from your senior resident.

- **Chest physiotherapy:** The patient with a collapsed lobe, significant atelectasis, or lobar pneumonia will benefit from chest physiotherapy.

- **Antibiotics:** If the patient appears to have a developing pneumonia, early antimicrobial treatment is important. Start broad-spectrum coverage if you believe it to be a hospital-acquired pneumonia.

- **Subcutaneous epinephrine:** If a patient appears to have signs of anaphylaxis, treat early with subcutaneous epinephrine, histamine blockers, and steroids.

37 Tachycardia

Jeremy Goodman

- **Crash cart location**
- **Hemodynamic instability?**
- **Signs of end-organ perfusion**
- **Chest pain or shortness of breath?**
- **Oxygen**
- **ECG**
- **Electrolytes**
- **CBC**
- **Chest x-ray**
- **IV access**

There's nothing like a patient with tachycardia to start your own heart racing. A mildly elevated heart rate may signify nothing more than inadequate pain control. At its extremes, however, tachycardia can be rapidly fatal. A heart rate >150 is rarely benign. This chapter assumes a familiarity with basic arrhythmia interpretation. Subtleties of ECG interpretation are not necessarily crucial; determine the rhythm and fix the problem.

Unstable tachycardia signifies a decrease in BP, ECG changes, or such signs of diminished end-organ perfusion as chest pain, shortness of breath, or altered mental status. These findings should lead to initiation of standard American Heart Association Advanced Cardiac Life Support (ACLS) protocols (see Appendix C). **Remember that first-line therapy for unstable tachycardia is electrical cardioversion.**

CHART REVIEW

- History of arrhythmia or other cardiac conditions
- History of cardiac surgery or pacemaker implantation

- Prehospital use of antiarrhythmics or rate-controlling medications
- Recent BP and heart rate trends
- Recent urine output trend

HISTORY

- Subjective sensation of palpitations, or "pounding heart"
- Chest pain, shortness of breath, or dizziness
- Any other pain, especially in the postoperative setting

PHYSICAL EXAM

- **Volume status:** Mucous membranes and skin turgor. Tachycardia is the first sign of volume depletion.
- **Cardiac exam:** Determine whether the rhythm is regular or irregular.

DIFFERENTIAL DIAGNOSIS

- **Sinus tachycardia**
  - Inadequate pain control
  - Volume depletion
  - Fever/infection
  - Anemia
  - Cardiac ischemia
  - Pulmonary embolism
  - Pneumothorax

- **Atrial flutter/fibrillation:** Commonly seen in elderly patients, especially those with a history of cardiac or pulmonary disease. Cardiac and thoracic operations increase the risk considerably. Volume overload is often associated. Atrial fibrillation may be considered rate controlled or non–rate controlled. A ventricular rate <100 in an asymptomatic patient is considered stable and controlled. Evaluate new-onset atrial fibrillation for an inciting event, such as pulmonary embolism, myocardial infarction, hyperthyroidism, or electrolyte abnormalities.

- **Paroxysmal supraventricular tachycardia:** Frequently triggered by severe pain; has a ventricular rate >150. Electrolyte abnormalities may contribute.

- **Ventricular tachycardia:** A true emergency, even when a pulse is present.

TESTING

- **ECG:** Critical in evaluating the patient with tachycardia. If there is some delay in finding a 12-lead machine, hook the patient up to the cardiac monitor on the code cart.

- **Cardiac labs:** Troponin-I or CK-MB.

- **Electrolytes:** Derangement of sodium, potassium, magnesium, calcium, or phosphorus can contribute.

- **ABG:** ABG will help support the diagnosis of pulmonary embolism. Also, extremes of pH can trigger arrhythmias.

- **V̇/Q̇ scan, CT scan, or angiogram:** To confirm pulmonary embolism. Check with your senior resident first.

TREATMENT

- Again, the treatment of specific life-threatening arrhythmias is systematically presented in the American Heart Association ACLS algorithms found in Appendix C. However, some general principles apply.

- **Oxygen:** Begin low-flow oxygen therapy until the tachycardia has resolved.

- **Cardiac monitoring:** Establish continuous cardiac monitoring. The frequency of vital sign measurements must be increased, which may necessitate transfer to an ICU.

- **Analgesia:** Adequately control pain, as this is a potent inducer of tachycardia. See Chap. 42, Pain, for more details.

- **Fluid bolus:** If volume depletion is suspected, give a 500- or 1000-mL normal saline bolus IV. Remember that the maintenance IV infusion rate may also need to be increased.

If atrial fibrillation is confirmed and the rate controlled, consider the long-term consequences of this arrhythmia. After approximately 72 hrs, thrombus can begin to form in the atria, predisposing to systemic embolization. If the rhythm does not spontaneously convert to sinus in that time period, the patient can be electively cardioverted. Alternatively, anticoagulation may be initiated.

38 Diet Status

Jeremy Goodman

You will frequently receive calls from the nurses to clarify a patient's diet status. These calls are usually prompted by the patient's request for food.

- If you are not familiar with the patient's hospital admission and course, be careful when initiating diet changes.

- NPO status is usually issued for a good reason. If a patient is NPO for a procedure or test, make sure it has been completed before resuming the diet. Remember that some patients will be scheduled for multiple tests in a single day. Check the chart to see if the patient can resume eating.

- You may be asked if a patient can eat food brought from home or the hospital cafeteria. In general, patients on a regular diet can eat homemade or favorite foods. Discourage patients on any kind of dietary restriction from eating outside foods.

- Requests to advance a patient's diet are generally addressed during rounds. If a patient on a liquid diet tolerates it well and has evidence of bowel function, it is usually safe to advance him or her to a solid diet. Note that this may not apply to patients after head and neck, upper GI, or bariatric (weight-reduction) surgery.

- See Part VIII on Nutrition for more detail.

39

Falls

Nirmal K. Veeramachaneni

Patients fall; people fall. Anywhere else, they would get up and get back in bed. In a hospital, it is a whole different matter. Patients, family, and caregivers will be very upset, and you will be called to make sure all is well.

Patients fall for a number of reasons. Your job is to differentiate the pathologic from the benign.

PHYSICAL EXAM

- Once you have made certain that the vital signs are stable, begin the secondary survey.

- Take great care in moving the patient. Perform logrolling and cervical immobilization to ensure that injuries are not worsened.

- Neurologic and musculoskeletal exams are mandatory. Focus attention on the cervical spine and palpate for tenderness before moving the neck. Also assess for other injuries.

- Once you have completed the above exams, consider obtaining orthostatic vital signs.

DIFFERENTIAL DIAGNOSIS

- **Neurologic:** Seizure, stroke, TIA

- **Delirium:** Metabolic, hypoxia, hypoglycemia, substance withdrawal, infection, psychosis

- **Cardiovascular:** Vasovagal episode, hypotension from multiple causes

- **Lines/tubes/drains:** As walking hazards

- **Drugs:** Narcotics, sedatives (overdose or withdrawal)

- **Postoperative weakness:** Anesthetic agents

- **Pain**

EVALUATION AND TREATMENT

- Check glucose and oxygen saturations. In an alert, oriented, and awake patient with a benign exam, no additional studies are required.

- Determine further investigation by the history obtained from the patient and the clinical scenario. Further evaluation may consist of cardiac enzymes and ECG, CBC for anemia or as a marker of infection, electrolytes, radiographic studies to assess for fracture or stroke, and ABG.

- Knowledge of the medical history, such as seizure disorder, poorly controlled diabetes, dementia, and medications, will clarify the situation.

- Treatment depends on the clinical problem.

- In a medically cleared patient who may have fallen due to confusion, consider a sitter in the room to supervise the patient and prevent further injury.

- Institute fall precautions (e.g., supervised ambulation, bed rails up). Restraints may be used, but with caution.

- Remember to document the circumstances of the situation and your findings. A patient's falling usually means an incident report to Risk Management, and therefore your medical documentation is essential.

40

Insomnia

Emily R. Winslow

The hospital environment is not conducive to sleep. Patients will frequently request a pill to help them get to sleep at night. Although it is tempting to give a sleeping pill to any patient who requests it, it is not always prudent.

Consider the following factors when thinking about administering a "sleeper":

- Patient age: Older patients can react poorly to most sleep-inducing medications, particularly benzodiazepines. They can become confused and disoriented, which is certainly worse than their not getting enough sleep. In general, we suggest avoiding sleeping pills for older patients. The only exception is in patients who take one routinely at home and know their medication name and dose. If you do give a new medication to older patients, do so cautiously and warn them of potential side effects.

- Pulmonary function: Most sleeping pills will depress respiratory drive to some extent. Patients with underlying pulmonary disease (COPD, emphysema, obstructive sleep apnea) and those who have undergone thoracic surgery are at particularly high risk from this complication.

- Concomitant medications: Most surgical patients receive some form of parenteral narcotic for pain. Benzodiazepines act synergistically with narcotics. Thus, even a small dose can have significant effects in a patient receiving IV narcotics.

- Reason for request: Even though it seems obvious why the patient is requesting a medication, the real problem may be something other than insomnia. Often, the patient can't sleep because of uncontrolled pain, the need for frequent urination, a loud roommate, a hallway light, or a loud nursing station. These problems should not be solved by administering a potentially dangerous medication. Do the right thing for your patient, even if it is not as easy as writing a quick order. Instead, helping to arrange a room transfer, turning off lights, or placing a Foley will generate better results.

If you decide to give the appropriate patient a sleeping pill, carefully consider which pill to give. The available classes are basically benzodiazepines (and benzo-like medications) and histamine antagonists.

Examples of frequently used medications include diphenhydramine (Benadryl), 25–50 mg IV/PO; temazepam (Restoril), 15–30 mg PO; triazolam (Halcion), 0.125 mg PO; and zolpidem tartrate (Ambien), 5–10 mg PO.

If you decide not to give a patient a sleeping pill, explain to the patient why you are not able to honor the request. Patients are frequently understanding if you take a minute to explain your concerns about side effects.

41

Lost IV Access

Emily R. Winslow

The fundamental issue in considering a lost IV is safety. If a patient does not have an indwelling IV line in place, delivery of IV medications and fluid is impossible. Your first job when called about a lost IV is to clarify whether the patient in fact needs one. If so, reestablish access either peripherally or centrally.

DOES THE PATIENT NEED AN IV?

- Almost all surgical patients need an IV while in the hospital.

- There are some exceptions. Patients who are eating and drinking, not receiving IV medications, and clinically stable may be able to avoid having an IV replaced. The most common example is the patient who is to be discharged within the next 24 hrs.

- Patients who are within the first 48 hrs of their postoperative course (unless the operation was minor) should always have an IV.

- Make sure your patient does not have an accessible Port-A-Cath or indwelling central line before deciding to replace an IV.

- You should never access hemodialysis catheters, except in emergencies.

WHAT KIND OF ACCESS DOES THE PATIENT NEED?

Once you have determined that your patient indeed needs IV access, decide whether he or she needs peripheral or central access.

- Central access is needed in patients on TPN, patients who need measurement of central venous pressure, patients receiving certain medications (e.g., pressors, some chemotherapy), and patients who need frequent blood draws and have exhausted their peripheral access.

- Most patients need only peripheral access.

How Do I Establish a Peripheral IV?

Most interns feel that if the nurse (especially the IV nurse) cannot establish a peripheral IV, it cannot be established. *This is absolutely not true*. Any time you are faced with this problem, you must assess the peripheral veins yourself.

- At a minimum, you must look for available veins. You will be surprised at the number of times you will succeed.

- Before placing an IV, make sure you know how large an IV is needed. If the patient is to receive a blood transfusion, you need a minimum of an 18-gauge IV.

- When looking for peripheral IV sites, first examine the hands and arms. Avoid the antecubital veins when possible, as these cause patient discomfort and restrict arm movement.

- Remember that in some patients, one extremity may not be available for IV placement owing to comorbid conditions (e.g., dialysis patients with grafts, postmastectomy patients).

- If the arms do not yield any possible sites, the next options are the external jugular veins. You should look at these veins on both sides of the neck with the patient in the Trendelenburg position. Note that these are peripheral veins, not central veins.

- In select circumstances, a lower-extremity IV may provide temporary peripheral access.

- If none of these sites looks promising, you will likely need to proceed to central access.

Establishing a Central Line

- Before deciding to establish central access, discuss the situation with a senior resident and get the patient's consent.

- If you have not had adequate training or do not feel comfortable placing a central line, call for help. See Appendix A, Procedures, for details.

42

Pain

Emily R. Winslow

Pain is the one symptom that all surgical patients share. But ordering a dose of morphine in response to every call about a patient in pain is not adequate patient care.

EVALUATE THE PATIENT

- Take a brief history.
- Check the vital signs.
- Examine the operative site.
- Assess the amount and type of medication the patient has received so far.
- Look for cocontributors to the pain.

DETERMINE THE CAUSE

Although it may seem obvious that pain is from the operative incision, that is not always the case. At times, pain can be secondary to a postoperative complication, such as intraabdominal bleeding. Other potential etiologies include

- Ineffective delivery of prior pain medication [infiltrated IV, patient-controlled analgesia (PCA) not available, misplaced epidural].
- Tolerance to narcotics (e.g., drug users and alcoholics).
- Complications (bleeding, missed diagnosis).
- Local problems (tight-fitting dressing, patient malposition, Foley catheter).

DETERMINE THE SEVERITY

Ask the patient to rate the pain on a scale from 1 to 10, with 10 being the most severe pain. Follow this over time so you will know how effective your interventions have been. Also assess the vital signs to see if the patient is tachycardic.

TREAT THE PAIN

There are many different ways to treat pain, but the most important objective is to initiate treatment promptly. Consider the following when deciding what medication to deliver:

Method of delivery:

- Intermittent IV dosing by nurse
- PCA
- Local delivery of anesthesia (epidural, local blocks)
- IM delivery
- PO medications

Type of medication:

- Narcotics
- Local anesthetics
- NSAIDs
- Acetaminophen

Patient comorbidities:

- Renal failure
- Hepatic insufficiency
- Patient age
- Bleeding potential

There is no one specific way to treat pain, but here are some general guidelines to get you started:

- Start with an IV narcotic in a dose that is appropriate for the patient's age, size, and pain severity. Usually, this means morphine in 2- to 4-mg doses. In the elderly, start with $1/2$ mg.
- In the patient with renal failure or hepatic insufficiency, carefully select narcotics. The best choices are fentanyl (Sublimaze) and hydromorphone (Dilaudid). In renal failure, accumulated metabolites of meperidine (Demerol) will lower the seizure threshold.
- Give NSAIDs judiciously because of their renal and platelet side effects. However, a parenteral dose of ketorolac (Toradol) can be a miraculous thing to the postoperative patient in pain.
- Patients who have a PCA but have ongoing pain are difficult to deal with. You need to assess the degree of narcotization (pupil size, respiratory rate) and their understanding of how to use the PCA. If they have been getting the maximum dosage and are not "over-narcotized," then the appropriate move is to give them several extra doses until they are comfortable and then to increase the dose of the PCA (not decrease the interval). It is unwise to give a basal rate on PCA in most situations.

- Patients who are refractory to narcotics and NSAIDs but who have substantial pain are good candidates to consider for an epidural placement. Call your pain or anesthesia team to help in this decision. If pain control is inadequate in patients with preoperative epidurals, test the epidural to make sure it is positioned properly.

- Consider giving PO pain medications when the pain is not severe and the patient tolerates PO intake. Giving PO pain medications to patients who are not eating will often lead to nausea and vomiting.

ASSESS THE RESPONSE TO THERAPY

After treating an acute episode of pain, you should later assess for over-narcotization and effective pain control. Finally, the most important aspect of reassessing the patient is to make sure the patient understands that you are an ally in terms of fighting the pain. Too often, patients feel that they have been left to suffer and that no one is concerned about their discomfort.

CONSULTATION

If your institution has a pain service (usually run by the anesthesia department), ask for help with chronic pain patients and those who do not respond as expected to standard analgesic regimens.

43 "Patient Doesn't Look Right"

Nirmal K. Veeramachaneni

These are dreaded words. Over the telephone, they provide no information. The bottom line: ***Go see the patient.*** Answers you get over the telephone will determine the speed at which you go to the bedside.

- As vital signs are vital, ask for them immediately. Go over the ABCs with the nurse. Is the patient awake or obtunded; is the patient responsive; is the patient breathing with normal vital signs? This basic triage information can easily be obtained over the telephone and guides the rapidity of your arrival at the bedside.

- When an experienced nurse calls, these words imply that the patient is sick, and a physician needs to be at the bedside. When an inexperienced nurse calls, the words mean the nurse has no idea what is going on and needs a physician to evaluate the patient.

- Once at the bedside, use the standard approach of the ABCs, look at the chart, and follow the vital sign trends.

- Think about the comorbid conditions and the potential complications of the procedure performed.

- The patients we treat are getting older and sicker. New problems constantly arise. For example, it would not be unheard of for an 80-yr-old to have a stroke after a cholecystectomy; 80-yr-olds have strokes.

- Once you are satisfied that the patient is stable, and a physical exam confirms your findings, immediately inform your senior resident and continue close observation.

44

Pharmacy Questions

Jeremy Goodman

Calls from the pharmacy will be initiated by illegible handwriting, dosing errors, or drug interactions. Although they may sometimes seem a nuisance, remember that the pharmacist has your patients' best interests at heart.

- *Write legibly*. Pharmacy orders are often sent by fax, and bad handwriting is only made worse by the transmission. If your orders are being transcribed or entered by a ward clerk or secretary, remember that he or she usually has no medical knowledge and little ability to creatively interpret your scribbles.

- Dosing errors are common. Remember that many medications must be adjusted for weight, renal and hepatic impairment, and severity of illness. The pharmacist can help you with these calculations.

- It is difficult to remember every possible drug interaction. The pharmacy department is vigilant in this respect and has an up-to-date record of each patient's current medications. Take their warnings seriously, and listen to suggestions for possible drug substitutions. *When in doubt, ask the pharmacist.*

45 Wound Drainage

Jeremy Goodman

Wound problems are common postoperatively and range from mild drainage to overt dehiscence. Additionally, wounds may become infected, and careful inspection should be a part of every postoperative patient's physical exam.

- Postoperative "spotting" of a dressing may be the result of intraoperative irrigation. Thicker or bloody drainage is more concerning. A small amount of postoperative bleeding is not uncommon and is most often the result of subcutaneous bleeding that will stop spontaneously. Nurses will often circle the stain on the bandage early on as a means of judging its spread over time.

- Thin or serous drainage can usually be left alone. When a dressing becomes soaked and must be replaced, it should be done under sterile conditions. Increased clear drainage and soaked dressings may reflect dehiscence of an abdominal closure.

- Bleeding from a wound should be closely monitored. It can reflect serious intraabdominal hemorrhage or merely minor bleeding from a subcutaneous source. If the bleeding continues or the patient becomes hemodynamically unstable, a CBC should be sent to assess the magnitude of blood loss. A PT and PTT may be requested if there is concern for coagulopathy. In some instances, a patient may need reoperation to treat bleeding.

- Wound drainage that begins several days postoperatively is infection until proven otherwise. Other local signs of infection include erythema, pain, and fluctuance. If the drainage point can be localized, the wound is often opened at this site by removing a few staples or sutures. The wound can then be probed to assess the extent of infection. Subcutaneous fluid collections should generally not be cultured, as contaminating skin flora make interpretation difficult. Wound infections are most often caused by gram-positive bacteria. Start patients on appropriate antibiotics and pack the wound with a dressing; allow it to heal by secondary intention.

- A subcutaneous fluid collection may be the result of fat necrosis, especially in obese patients. This type of drainage is thin and yellow to clear, and often demonstrates fat droplets in the fluid. Treatment includes opening the wound and packing.

- Fascial dehiscence is the separation of the deepest layers of the abdominal wound. This condition is an emergency, and prompt recognition and surgical treatment may help limit the possibility of evisceration in abdominal wounds.

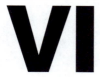

VI

Common Problems

. . . look for horses, not zebras . . .

Throughout this book, we have tried to provide general information as it pertains to the surgical patient. You will quickly learn, however, that each type of procedure carries specific risks and complications. Unfortunately, a list of every general surgical procedure is beyond the scope of this book. Here, we consider broad surgical categories and organ systems, highlighting specific concerns for each. What follows is by no means a comprehensive list, but rather a brief look at the most common issues.

46

Breast

Nirmal K. Veeramachaneni

DRAINS

- Drains are usually left in place if a tissue flap (e.g., after mastectomy) is created. Pay attention to their proper function, as an undrained fluid collection may become infected.

- Some surgeons prefer to continue antibiotics until all of the drains have been removed.

- Postoperative evaluation should also focus on the integrity of the skin flaps. Flaps that are too thin may become cyanotic, ischemic, and eventually necrotic.

AXILLARY DISSECTION

- Axillary dissection may lead to injury to nerves and vessels. During postoperative evaluation, document intact axillary nerves (long thoracic nerve injury results in serratus anterior paralysis and "winged scapula," and thoracodorsal nerve injury results in latissimus dorsi weakness).

- Paresthesias in the axilla may be due to intercostobrachial nerve injury.

- A postoperative exercise regimen can help with swelling and diminished mobility.

SENTINEL NODE BIOPSY

- Sentinel node biopsy has the peculiar complication of discolored urine. The vital blue dye is excreted by the kidneys. Reassure patients.

47 Esophagus and Upper GI

Emily R. Winslow

NASOGASTRIC TUBE MANIPULATION

- In patients undergoing esophageal or upper GI surgery, the NG tube is placed in the OR under direct visualization. Surgery on the esophagus and stomach disrupts the anatomy to such an extent that blind NG tube placement is difficult and potentially dangerous. All such patients should have a sign placed over the bed that says, "Do Not Manipulate NG Tube."

- If the NG tube becomes hopelessly clogged or even dislodged, check with a senior resident before replacing it blindly.

REPLACING OUTPUT

- Any patient with an NG tube can lose significant fluid and electrolytes in the aspirate, especially after upper GI surgery. If the patient is becoming dehydrated or if the electrolytes are altered, replace the NG tube output. The fluid can be replaced IV mL for mL or with a smaller ratio if volume overload is a concern.

  - If the NG output is primarily stomach contents, use 0.45% normal saline with supplemental potassium ($1/2$ normal saline + 20 mEq KCl/L).

  - For bilious output, use lactated Ringers to replace the bicarbonate-rich fluid.

SWALLOWING

- After esophageal and stomach surgery, the swallowing mechanism may be disrupted. These patients should follow strict aspiration precautions. The head of the bed should be elevated at least 30 degrees at all times and fluid and meals ingested in an upright position.

DRAINS

- Monitor neck drains carefully after esophageal surgery.

- An anastomotic leak can have serious consequences and may be detected early by a change in the quantity or quality of drainage.

48 General Abdominal Surgery

Emily R. Winslow

When examining patients who have had major open intraabdominal operations, you will notice that many are distended and complain of feeling "bloated." This is not at all unusual for the first several days postoperatively and usually improves within 4–5 days, depending on both the nature of the preoperative pathology and the extent of the operative procedure. However, some patients have an increased degree or extended duration of postoperative distention. The following are key aspects of the different processes that may be responsible.

PARALYTIC ILEUS

- Nontoxic patient with complaints of only distention and sometimes nausea and vomiting.

- Some improvement with conservative measures.

- Slowly resolving over time; not worsening.

- Abdominal x-ray shows nonspecific bowel gas pattern, mildly distended small and large bowel, scattered air-fluid levels.

PARTIAL SMALL BOWEL OBSTRUCTION

- Nausea, vomiting, and some degree of abdominal discomfort.

- No improvement with conservative measures, except possibly NG tube placement.

- Waxing and waning course, not necessarily improving.

- Abdominal x-ray shows air fluid levels, a suggestion of a transition point, and bowel wall thickening.

COMPLETE SMALL BOWEL OBSTRUCTION

- Worsening abdominal pain, nausea, vomiting, and possibly fever.

- Conservative measures aren't effective.

- Distention worsens with time.

- Abdominal x-ray shows marked distention, air-fluid levels or a gasless abdomen, suggestion of a transition point, and loss of the psoas sign.

MANAGEMENT
CT Scan

- Depending on how ill the patient appears, an abdominal/pelvic CT scan may be ordered if the plain film suggests a possible mechanical problem. *Check with a senior resident before ordering a CT scan.*

- The issue of PO contrast is a difficult one in patients with possible bowel obstructions. Attempt to give all patients water-soluble contrast before the CT scan, as this will help delineate where the problem is. This can be done via NG tube if the patient will not tolerate PO liquids.

- The timing of the contrast in relation to the scan is critical. It is best to give some contrast 1–2 hrs before and then to give a second, smaller bolus immediately before the scan. The CT scan will give a clearer picture of the obstruction level by the location of the ingested contrast.

Conservative Approach

Patients with an ileus will improve. Things that will help speed their recovery are maximizing ambulation, decreasing narcotics and other medications that slow intestinal motility, correcting electrolytes, and delaying diet advancement. Be patient and wait for the nausea and distention to resolve, and then advance the diet as usual.

Symptom Relief

Place an NG tube for symptom relief. Patients with persistent nausea and vomiting are miserable. Giving antiemetics does not improve a mechanical problem.

Fluid Status

Follow fluid status closely in patients with small bowel obstructions. They may need replacement of their NG output with IV fluid and should have their urine output assessed on a frequent basis.

Electrolytes and Renal Function

Assess daily.

Management Plan

Develop with your senior resident. There are many different postoperative approaches to bowel obstructions. Things to consider:

- Getting a GI contrast study (small bowel follow through, hypaque enema) to rule out anastomotic problems as the cause of the obstruction.

- Proceeding directly to the OR for reexploration.

- Observing the patient for a limited amount of time to see in which direction the patient is heading, as partial small bowel obstructions may resolve spontaneously with time. See Chap. 54, Abdominal Observation Patients.

49 Herniorrhaphy

Jeremy Goodman

The two most common hernia repairs you will be involved with are inguinal and ventral abdominal. Today, the vast majority of inguinal herniorrhaphies are done on an outpatient basis. Small ventral or incisional hernia repairs may be performed in the ambulatory setting. Larger hernias necessitate an inpatient recovery.

URINARY RETENTION

- Urinary retention is not uncommon in men after inguinal herniorrhaphy.

- No man should be discharged after hernia repair without voiding first, especially in the outpatient setting, where close postoperative monitoring is not possible.

TESTICLE

- In men, traction on the spermatic cord during herniorrhaphy may displace the testicle from the scrotum. At the end of the procedure, replace the testicle into the scrotum with gentle traction.

- Warn your patients that inguinal and scrotal bruising is common.

ILEUS

- After repair of ventral abdominal hernias, a brief postoperative ileus is common.

- If a significant amount of intestine was contained in the hernia sac, your patient may wait several days for return of bowel function.

SEROMA

- After repair of large ventral hernias, especially laparoscopic repair, patients may develop seromas. Fluid collects in the space previously occupied by the hernia sac.

- If anticipated intraoperatively, a drain may be left in place.

- Seromas can usually be left to reabsorb on their own. If sizable, they may be sterilely drained at the bedside with a needle and syringe. Check with your senior resident before performing such a procedure.

50 Laparoscopy

Emily R. Winslow

PAIN

Unlike after open abdominal surgery, patients do not usually experience much pain after laparoscopic procedures.

Shoulder Pain

- After laparoscopic surgery, many patients complain of shoulder pain. This is referred pain and is secondary to unabsorbed gas that is irritating the diaphragm. It should resolve with time.

- Relief of this pain is difficult. Ambulation often shifts the gas to a different position. NSAIDs and narcotics can be effective.

Abdominal Pain

- Any patient with severe abdominal pain after a laparoscopic procedure should be carefully examined, because it is very unusual and can point to a major operative complication. Things to consider are bowel injuries with peritonitis and intraabdominal bleeding.

- Pain after a laparoscopic gallbladder removal should alert you to a possible bile duct injury or biloma.

Chest Pain

- After laparoscopic surgery around the esophageal hiatus (e.g., Nissen, Toupet, Heller), be alert to the possibility of a "slipped wrap," a wrap that has migrated through the diaphragmatic hiatus into the chest. If detected in the early postoperative period, it is easily solved by returning to the OR. If diagnosis is delayed, reoperative surgery is much more difficult.

- Perforation, although uncommon, may also occur after esophageal manipulation.

PNEUMOTHORAX

- If your patient gets a chest x-ray after a laparoscopic procedure, you may note a pneumothorax.

- It may occur after esophageal hiatal surgery, in which the pleural membrane can be easily violated.

- It usually does not require intervention (unless the patient is symptomatic), as the CO_2 is rapidly reabsorbed.

SUBCUTANEOUS EMPHYSEMA

- Subcutaneous emphysema results from dissection of CO_2 into the subcutaneous plane at some point during the surgery. It resolves without intervention and is usually not a cause for alarm.

- However, you must consider other possibilities in patients at risk. For example, esophageal perforation after bougie insertion may lead to pneumomediastinum and subcutaneous emphysema.

HYDROCELE

After pelvic laparoscopic procedures such as hernia repairs and node dissections, patients may develop a hydrocele. This is the result of irrigation fluid accumulation in the most dependent areas. It will resolve spontaneously as the patient begins to ambulate.

51

Liver/Pancreas/ Gallbladder

Emily R. Winslow and Jeremy Goodman

BILIARY LEAKS AND BILOMA

- After biliary surgery, bile leakage from the wound should be investigated promptly. It is easily recognized in the wound by its typical green color.

- A *biloma* refers to a walled-off collection of bile within the abdominal cavity.

- Bile leaks and bilomas often need prompt intervention to prevent secondary infection.

- The range of management options includes endoscopic retrograde cholangiopancreatography (ERCP) and stenting, transhepatic biliary drain placement, intraabdominal drain placement, and reoperation.

BILE DUCT INJURY

- Since the introduction of laparoscopic cholecystectomy, more attention has been paid to the complication of bile duct injuries. Bile duct injury is trauma to a duct other than the cystic duct, usually occurring during a laparoscopic cholecystectomy.

- Several typical patterns of ductal injuries occur, but all involve devascularization or clipping of a duct (often the common bile duct).

- It can be discovered during the course of the initial operation, but more commonly the diagnosis is delayed until the patient develops symptoms of biliary obstruction. Pain, fevers, and vomiting are typical symptoms and need to be investigated promptly.

- Management principles include immediate referral to an experienced hepatobiliary surgeon, initiation of antibiotics, and drainage of any blocked segments of the biliary tree (either via ERCP or transhepatic biliary drain placement).

PANCREATIC INJURY AND PANCREATITIS

- After any surgery in the pancreatic region, pancreatic injury can result. It can manifest as a *pancreatic leak*, which refers to the presence of pancreatic fluid outside the ductal system.

- A pancreatic leak is a problem because of the digestive properties of pancreatic fluid, which cause significant tissue trauma.

- Pancreatitis can also result from blunt trauma to the pancreas in the course of an operation.

- Having a high index of suspicion for these problems is crucial. If you suspect a pancreatic leak and an intraoperative drain has been placed, check the amylase level of the fluid. For pancreatitis, check the serum amylase and lipase.

COAGULOPATHY

- After large liver resections, the body's ability to make clot may be significantly compromised. The remaining liver will need to produce an adequate amount of clotting factors, and in the immediate postoperative catabolic state, this is often not possible. Checking the PT serially after a liver resection is prudent, as these patients are at high risk of bleeding.

- FFP should be given as needed to keep the PT within an acceptable range. In addition, serial CBCs are essential to rule out postoperative bleeding from the raw liver edge.

52

Lower GI

Nirmal K. Veeramachaneni

URINARY RETENTION

- Urinary retention is a very common problem after any form of pelvic surgery.

- Poorly controlled pain after hemorrhoid surgery may also lead to urinary retention.

- Placement of a Foley catheter usually solves the problem.

- To avoid urinary retention, some surgeons recommend continuing the catheter for several days after such procedures as abdominoperineal resection.

BOWEL HABIT CHANGES

It may take months for bowel habits to normalize after colon surgery. See Chaps. 29 and 30, Constipation and Diarrhea, for more information.

HEMORRHOID SURGERY

- Hemorrhoid surgery is performed by either ligation of the varices or excision.

- Complications include pain, secondary thrombosis of external hemorrhoids, and sepsis.

- Increasing pain, fever, and urinary retention may herald pelvic sepsis.

53

Nirmal K. Veeramachaneni

AIRWAY

Any evidence of dysphonia or stridor should prompt rapid evaluation and intervention. Do not hesitate to intubate the patient if indicated. The obstruction may be at one of multiple levels:

- **Oropharynx:** In the overweight patient with a short, fat neck, obtaining airway access may be challenging. Even an experienced anesthesiologist may have significant difficulty with intubation. Multiple attempts may lead to swelling and inflammation of the oropharynx. Treatment with steroids or nebulized racemic epinephrine may help.

- **Larynx:** Inflammation of the cords due to trauma, anaphylaxis, or nerve injury (see Nerve Injury) may lead to compromise.

- **Tracheal/bronchial:** After surgery in the mouth, fluid and blood may accumulate in the airways. A poor cough reflex will lead to mucus plugging and poor air movement. Preoperative COPD may include a significant reactive airway component. Chest physiotherapy, nebulizer treatments, and bronchoscopy (as a last resort) may help. Have the patient out of bed if possible.

VESSELS

- The neck is a very vascular region, and bleeding is not unusual. For this reason, drains are frequently left in place.

- A hematoma may become infected, cause significant discomfort, or even cause airway compromise.

LYMPHATICS

- Diagnose persistent lymphatic drainage by measuring triglyceride levels in the effluent. Diet restriction can help seal the leak. Operative intervention may be required for persistent leak.

NERVE INJURY

- **Mandibular branch of the facial nerve:** Ipsilateral drooping of the corner of the mouth and drooling.

- **Hypoglossal nerve:** Deviation of the tongue toward the side of injury and difficulty with speech and swallowing.

- **Recurrent laryngeal nerve:** Vocal cord paralysis, hoarseness, and loss of effective cough mechanism. Bilateral nerve injury may lead to complete vocal cord paralysis, necessitating tracheostomy.

- **Superior laryngeal nerve:** Easy fatigability of voice, inability to phonate high-pitched notes.

- **Greater auricular nerve:** Numbness or painful paresthesia of the earlobe and scalp.

THYROID GLAND

After a cancer operation, thyroid replacement is typically held to induce a state of hypothyroidism. Elevated TSH facilitates radioactive iodine ablation.

PARATHYROID GLAND

Hypocalcemia is caused by hypoparathyroidism. Symptoms include paresthesia of the mouth and fingers, Chvostek's sign (facial twitches with gentle percussion of the facial nerve as it traverses the parotid gland), and Trousseau's sign (carpal spasm with flexion of the wrist during BP cuff compression of the arm).

- Asymptomatic hypocalcemia usually does not require treatment.

- Symptoms necessitate PO or IV calcium, depending on their severity. Vitamin D supplements may also be given.

- In the event of reimplantation of the parathyroid glands, transient hypocalcemia is almost certain.

- Similarly, resection for secondary hyperparathyroidism often leaves the patient with bone hunger; the sudden decrease in parathyroid hormone leads to reabsorption of calcium by bone and hypocalcemia.

54

Abdominal Observation Patients

Emily R. Winslow

Although most surgical patients come with a known diagnosis for a specific operation, sometimes patients are admitted to a surgical service with an unclear picture. These patients are usually admitted for "observation" from the ER. A typical scenario is a patient with abdominal pain of unclear etiology who is too sick to go home but too well to warrant an operation. The situation leaves the surgical intern in a quandary, as these patients fit into none of our usual categories.

WRITING THE ORDERS

When writing orders for observation patients, remember that their trajectory is unclear. In 8 hrs, they may be ready for discharge, or, alternatively, they may be in the OR. Always act with this in mind.

- **Keep all patients NPO** unless your senior resident has directed you otherwise.

- **Give liberal maintenance IV fluids.** Any patient with nausea or vomiting needs adequate hydration.

- **Don't write for routine pain medications.** Do not order routine analgesics for these patients unless there is a compelling reason to do so. Instead, write an order for the nurse to call you for a complaint of pain. You should always examine these patients before giving additional pain medications, as pain complaints may signal an important change in patient status.

- **If infection is a concern,** it is appropriate to recheck a CBC the morning after admission to see in which direction the WBC count is trending.

- Consider ordering a **type and screen** if this has not been done already.

- **Patient temperature:** Write a specific order for the nursing staff to call you for any elevation in patient temperature. Remember, these patients have fevers secondary to real pathology, not "routine low-grade postoperative fevers" or "atelectasis."

- **Order "ins and outs"** as with other patients. Low urine output points to a significant problem and will help you gauge the severity of a patient's illness.

EXAMINING THE PATIENT

The most important task in taking care of the observation patient is performing careful serial exams. To do this well, you need to do a deliberate and careful initial evaluation.

- **Take a brief history.** Hear for yourself how the patient describes the symptoms and their intensity.

- **Perform a careful abdominal exam.** Assess for any diffuse or localized peritonitis. Get a sense for how severe the pain is with gentle palpation. Assess for any masses. Look carefully for scars to indicate prior operations that may have been missed in the ER.

WHAT TO DO NEXT

The patient admitted for observation has been admitted to be **observed by you.** This is a *significant* responsibility that you should take seriously.

- Perform serial abdominal exams throughout the night. Depending on the severity and nature of the patient's complaints, you need to examine the patient q2–4h. You should plan to visit the patient's room throughout the night. Do so faithfully and carefully. Going into a patient's room at 4 a.m. to awaken and examine him or her can seem like overkill to a busy intern. It is essential that you do it anyway. Document each exam.

- Reassess the patient with any change in symptoms. If the nurse calls you, even with a seemingly minor complaint (e.g., nausea), briefly see the patient and reassess for any significant changes. Remember, you are the one responsible for *observing* the observation patient.

WHEN TO CALL FOR HELP

Should the patient appear to be rapidly evolving from somewhat well to rather sick, let your senior know. The patient may need operative intervention. Waiting until morning rounds to tell your senior resident about a change in the patient's condition is always a bad idea.

55

Spleen

Nirmal K. Veeramachaneni

IMMUNIZATION

- Asplenic individuals are prone to infections by encapsulated organisms.
- Ideally, patients should receive immunization against *Pneumococcus, Haemophilus influenzae B,* and *Meningococcus* several weeks before the operation. In the event that this is not possible (e.g., trauma), perform immunization before the patient leaves the hospital.

BLEEDING

- Blood products and platelets should be available, especially if hypersplenism is the indication for splenectomy.
- A type and cross (not type and screen) is necessary in any patient having splenectomy with a high likelihood of having antibodies. These antibodies make it more difficult and time-consuming for the blood bank to crossmatch a compatible unit of blood. This is best done the day before operation.

PANCREATIC INJURY

- Pancreatic injury is possible owing to the anatomic association of the tail of the pancreas to the splenic hilum.
- Pancreatic injury is indicated by abdominal pain, effusion, and amylase and lipase elevation.

INFECTION

- Postsplenectomy leukocytosis may hide true underlying infection.
- Overwhelming postsplenectomy sepsis syndrome has an incidence of approximately 4% with a mortality rate of 1.7%.
- Subtle signs of infection should prompt treatment with antibiotics.

THROMBOEMBOLISM

- Postsplenectomy elevation in leukocytes and platelets is common, and this may play a role in the thromboembolic phenomenon (i.e., DVT, pulmonary embolism) to which these patients are especially susceptible.
- Antiplatelet agents (aspirin) are begun for counts >1 million.

56 Trauma

Jeremy Goodman

SECONDARY SURVEY

In the excitement of the initial resuscitation, non–life-threatening injuries can be overlooked. For the patient in extremis, there may not be time for a thorough and complete secondary survey in the ER. Therefore, it is your job to carefully examine all trauma patients when they arrive on the ward.

- Pay careful attention to the scalp, back, perineum, fingers, and toes. These are the most frequently overlooked areas.

CERVICAL SPINE INJURIES

- Most centers require both radiographic and clinical clearance of cervical spine injuries before the protective collar is removed. Before removing a cervical collar, confirm that radiographic studies are negative. Look at the films yourself.

- A sober patient without distracting, painful injuries may be clinically cleared by removing the collar and palpating for bony tenderness along the cervical spine. Next, have the patient flex and rotate the neck. Pain or paresthesia is an indication to immediately stop the test, reapply the collar, and obtain additional imaging studies (e.g., flexion and extension views of the cervical spine).

ER STUDIES

Often, numerous radiographic studies are ordered in the ER evaluation of the trauma patient.

- Make sure the results of every test are appropriately documented in the chart. Never take someone's word for it; if in doubt, find out the results yourself.

- In the middle of the night, a preliminary interpretation may be the only one available. Make sure to follow up on official reports the next day.

TOXICOLOGY

Trauma victims may also be users or abusers of alcohol or illegal drugs.

- Many trauma centers include blood and urine toxicology in their standard lab panel. Some of these tests take hours to run, and results may become available only after the patient has been transferred to your care.

- See if your institution has an optional or mandatory counseling program for drug and alcohol users.

- Remember to never discuss the results of toxicology studies with anyone other than the medical team and patient.

SOCIAL ISSUES

Social problems often follow the trauma patient into the hospital.

- The homeless trauma patient will need arrangements for shelter and discharge medications. Get the social worker or case coordinator involved early on.

- Intoxicated patients may demand to be discharged once sober. If you believe the patient is competent and able to understand the consequence of his or her actions, you may not hold him.

- Patients under police custody should be dealt with in the presence of security or law enforcement personnel.

57

Vascular

Nirmal K. Veeramachaneni

PULSES

- Assessing for distal pulses should be part of the physical exam performed on every vascular patient. Note the presence or absence of pulses and their character.

- You can chart in table form or on a stick-figure diagram of the body.

- Assess the upper extremity at the brachial and radial arteries.

- The lower extremity includes the femoral, popliteal, dorsalis pedis, and posterior tibial arteries.

- Assess pulse manually, with your fingers, or auscultate it with the Doppler probe. Ultrasound jelly or water-based lubricant improves sound transmission with the probe.

- If you cannot find the pulse, check the chart to see if it has ever been documented as present. **A change in pulse status, especially distal to a revascularization, mandates an immediate call to your senior resident.**

COLD LIMB

- *A cold limb after vascular surgery is an emergency.*

- After revascularization, most extremities improve in color and increase in temperature. A cold limb suggests failure of the bypass, usually by thrombosis.

- Check carefully for pulses as discussed above.

- If the patient is immediately postoperative and suspicion is high, take him or her directly back to the OR for angiography and reexploration.

SWOLLEN LIMB

Virtually all limbs swell after vascular surgery.

- Minimize swelling by encouraging elevation of the affected extremity. Include an elevation order in the chart.

- Inform the patient that most swelling will resolve by 2–3 wks after surgery.

- Be sure to exclude deep venous thrombosis in these high-risk patients, however.

COMPARTMENT SYNDROME

If the pressure within an extremity exceeds capillary pressure, ischemia and compartment syndrome will result.

- Remember that absence of arterial pulses is a late sign of compartment syndrome. It may be diagnosed earlier by the presence of the five "Ps": paresthesia, pressure, pallor, pain, and poikilothermia (coolness).

- Traditionally, the pain of compartment syndrome is described as greatest with passive extension of the affected muscles.

- Direct measurement of a compartment pressure >30 mm Hg is diagnostic.

- Emergent fasciotomy is the only treatment.

COMORBIDITIES

The majority of vascular patients are elderly and have multiple comorbidities.

- Cardiac, pulmonary, and endocrinologic disturbances are common.

- Several recent studies advocate the use of preoperative beta-blockers in certain patients having vascular surgery; check with your senior resident or attending.

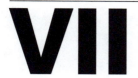

VII

Critical Care

. . . q1min vitals, please . . .

58

Crashing Patient

Nirmal K. Veeramachaneni

SICK OR NOT SICK?

Knowing which patients are truly sick is perhaps the junior resident's most difficult lesson.

- We often underestimate the patient's precarious condition. If the patient doesn't look right, the patient is probably *not* right.

- Through experience, you will develop an understanding of the patient's expected course. Deviation from that course should prompt investigation. For example, if patients normally eat after a Nissen fundoplication, but one patient complains of pain or lack of appetite, it is your responsibility to find out if something is wrong.

VITAL SIGNS ARE VITAL

- Never ignore an abnormal value. Abnormal vital signs are sentinels of impending catastrophe, so all abnormalities must be explained.

- Especially in the extremes of age, they offer subtle clues. Tachycardia may be the initial sign of a hematocrit of 20%!

MOBILIZING THE TROOPS

- When you perceive something to be abnormal, the first step should be to *call a senior resident*. No attending or senior resident will blame you for discussing low urine output (or other abnormal values) at 2 a.m. You will, however, be blamed at 7 a.m. if the abnormal finding was known only by you, and the appropriate treatment regimen was not followed.

- As the junior resident, your job is to recognize what is abnormal and alert the right person to discuss your treatment plan. *There is a failure of communication if the junior resident is the only one who knows that something is wrong.*

"CONCERNING" OR "EMERGENT"?

This question relates to the acuity of the condition. Address the ABCs and ensure IV access.

CAN I ADEQUATELY MONITOR THE PATIENT?

The patient may need central line monitoring, arterial BP monitoring, or a Foley catheter. Determine the tools you will need.

CAN I USE THESE TOOLS IN THE PRESENT SETTING?

- Having a Foley or a central line is useless if the nurse is not able to record frequent urine output or there is no monitor for continuous central venous pressure measurement. Knowing nursing policy and resources is crucial. Determine what the nursing needs are, and transfer the patient to an appropriate setting.

- As a general rule, don't fight nursing policy. If the charge nurse says he or she can't take care of the patient, move the patient!

CAN I DEAL WITH COMPLICATIONS?

This is an important question when there are impending cardiac or pulmonary events.

- Serious arrhythmias and respiratory failure are best dealt with in an ICU.

TRANSFERRING THE PATIENT TO THE ICU

- Call early, before the condition progresses from "concerning" to "emergent," and make sure a bed is available.

- When calling, present the patient to whoever is in charge of admitting patients to the ICU. Be prepared to present a short history: who the patient is, what comorbid diseases the patient has, and what complication you are attempting to treat.

- If the ICU is not willing to accept the patient, contact your senior resident or attending immediately. This is either a failure to communicate the gravity of the illness or to appreciate the severity of the illness. If you are unable to effectively make the case, let your senior do so.

- As the physical transfer is being arranged, complete the evaluation and initial treatment. Don't wait for the ICU team to draw the labs, place the Foley, or obtain IV access.

- Keep the patient continuously monitored, and transport the patient with a cardiac monitor. Keep airway access tools available during transport.

- On transferring the patient, be prepared to present the patient's history to the ICU team. They have never seen this patient before and will appreciate not having to immediately sort through a dense chart.

DOCUMENTATION

Your last task is to document the course of events in the chart. The transfer note should briefly recapitulate key aspects of the patient's history, events on the floor, treatment undertaken, and specific reasons for transfer.

Codes

59

Jeremy Goodman

The lesson is not to panic. Often, you will be the first physician at the scene. In a hospital, rest assured that reinforcements will arrive, and someone with more experience may be able to help direct care. Your job as the first physician on the scene is to ensure that the ABCs are evaluated and secured. Refer to the Appendixes for ACLS algorithms and a guide to procedures.

AIRWAY/BREATHING

- If you are unable to intubate, remember that alternative means of preserving the airway exist. The bag-valve device can effectively ventilate the patient if used in the proper manner.

- It may be difficult for a single rescuer to secure the mask and squeeze the bag; enlist help.

- Remember to place an oropharyngeal airway and tilt the patient's neck back into the sniffing position (if no contraindication exists).

- Cricoid pressure may be helpful.

- Always ensure that the chest is moving.

CIRCULATION

IV access is critical to proper resuscitation.

- The first instinct is to attempt a central line. This is often difficult, given the lack of a pulse to serve as a landmark and the motion of the patient due to CPR.

- Attempt to place a peripheral line first. Adequate delivery of agents can be achieved peripherally if each medication is followed by a bolus of carrier fluid.

- Remember that some agents, such as lidocaine, epinephrine, and atropine, may be given via the endotracheal tube when no IV access is available (give 2–2.5 times the IV dose in 10 mL saline).

COORDINATING CARE

Once reinforcements arrive, continue to assist in the resuscitation efforts. As the most junior member of the team, you will be the one most likely to know the patient's history.

• Find the chart and review the most recent labs. Knowing the medical history will help guide therapy.

• Call the ICU early in the resuscitation to alert them to a possible transfer.

60 Ventilators

Jeremy Goodman

Mechanical ventilators come in all shapes and sizes and can be programmed to deliver artificial breaths in a variety of ways. Broadly speaking, ventilatory strategies can be divided into two main categories: those that are volume controlled and those that are pressure controlled.

VOLUME-CONTROLLED VENTILATION

In volume-controlled ventilation, a tidal volume (often 6–10 mL/kg) is programmed, and the machine delivers this specific amount.

- The pressure generated is inversely proportional to the patient's lung compliance. In other words, a stiff lung causes a higher pressure to deliver the same volume of gas.

- Ventilators are equipped with a high-pressure alarm, and a maximum pressure limit may be set.

- Bear in mind that if the resulting pressure exceeds the set threshold, the breath may be prematurely terminated.

- This mode of ventilation is appropriate for most patients but may be harmful in the setting of decreased lung compliance, as in severe pneumonia or acute respiratory distress syndrome.

PRESSURE-CONTROLLED VENTILATION

In pressure-controlled ventilation, a driving pressure is programmed, and the machine delivers gas at that pressure over a specified duration of time.

- A specific tidal volume is not delivered; the volume of gas varies from breath to breath.

- As lung compliance decreases, so does the volume of gas delivered at a set pressure. This may lead to underventilation of the patient.

- This mode of ventilation may be used for any patient but is commonly reserved for situations in which volume control may lead to unacceptably high airway pressures, as in severe pneumonia or acute respiratory distress syndrome.

- When underventilation is expected and accepted, it is referred to as *permissive hypercapnia.*

ASSIST/CONTROL VENTILATION

Tidal volume and respiratory rate are set, and the machine delivers regardless of patient contribution. If the patient attempts a spontaneous breath, the machine is triggered to deliver an additional breath at the designated tidal volume.

INTERMITTENT MANDATORY VENTILATION

Tidal volume and respiratory rate are set, and the machine delivers regardless of patient contribution. Spontaneous breaths by the patient are unassisted, unless pressure support is added (see below). This mode may be *synchronized* so that machine-delivered breaths do not stack on top of spontaneous breaths.

POSITIVE END-EXPIRATORY PRESSURE (PEEP)

As the glottis closes on expiration in the nonintubated patient, air is trapped under pressure in the airways; this is called *physiologic PEEP*. It serves to keep the alveoli from completely collapsing, as they would if all the air were evacuated from them with each breath. The intubated patient loses physiologic PEEP, but it can be replaced by the ventilator. The commonly used minimum PEEP setting is 5 cm H_2O. As PEEP is increased, more alveoli are recruited, which can lead to improved oxygenation in the patient with impaired gas exchange. As PEEP, and consequently intrathoracic pressure, is increased, central venous blood return may be compromised. At high-enough levels, PEEP can impair cardiac function.

PRESSURE SUPPORT

With the addition of pressure support to volume-controlled ventilation, the ventilator assists each spontaneous breath that the patient takes. When the machine senses the patient's inspiratory effort, it delivers gas at the designated pressure to ease work of breathing. Set at a high-enough pressure support, the ventilator may provide 100% of the work of breathing.

FRACTION OF INSPIRED OXYGEN (Fio$_2$)

Fio_2 determines the concentration of oxygen in the inspired gas. Recall that room air contains 21% oxygen. An Fio_2 >80% should be avoided for prolonged periods of time owing to the risk of pulmonary and systemic oxygen toxicity.

61 Invasive Monitoring

Jeremy Goodman

ARTERIAL LINE

Used to continuously monitor BP and for arterial blood drawing.

CENTRAL VENOUS LINE

- Used to measure central venous pressure (CVP).

- The Cordis-type introducer sheath gives a more accurate measurement than does a multilumen catheter.

- The CVP trend may be more useful than the absolute number.

- This type of monitoring is useful in helping to determine a patient's volume status (preload).

PULMONARY ARTERY CATHETER (SWAN-GANZ)

- Directly measures CVP and pulmonary artery pressure.

- When the balloon at the tip is inflated, the pulmonary catheter wedge pressure is measured. In most situations, this provides an estimate of left atrial filling pressure and is one of the best means of assessing volume status.

- Also, a number of hemodynamic values (e.g., cardiac output, systemic vascular resistance) can be derived.

- These catheters are used when volume status and cardiac performance must be known.

62

Medications

Jeremy Goodman

The majority of cardiac and vasoactive drugs used in the ICU are exclusive to that setting. Tables 62-1 and 62-2 demonstrate the most common.

TABLE 62-1.
PROPERTIES OF VASOACTIVE DRUGS
COMMONLY USED IN THE ICU

	Alpha	Beta$_1$	Beta$_2$
Dobutamine	+	++++	++
Dopamine	++/+++	++++	++
Epinephrine	++++	++++	+++
Norepinephrine	++++	++++	+/++
Phenylephrine	++/+++	–	–

–, no activity; +, minimal activity; ++, mild activity; +++, moderate activity; ++++, maximum activity.
From Breslow MJ, Ligier B. Hyperadrenergic states. *Crit Care Med* 1991;19(12):1566–1579, with permission.

TABLE 62-2.
SUMMARY OF DRUGS COMMONLY USED IN THE ICU

Drug	Loading dose	Maintenance dose	Action	Side effects
Amiodarone	150 mg over 10 min	1 mg/min ×6 hr, then 0.5 mg/min	Class III antiarrhythmic	Hypotension, bradycardia
Diltiazem	0.25 mg/kg	5–15 mg/hr	Calcium channel blocker	Hypotension
Dobutamine	—	2–20 μg/kg/min	Beta agonist	Hypotension, tachycardia, arrhythmias
Dopamine	—	1–3 μg/kg/min: renal (dopaminergic) dose 3–10 μg/kg/min: beta (cardiac) dose >10 μg/kg/min: alpha (pressor) dose	Dopaminergic, beta, and alpha agonist	Tachycardia, arrhythmias
Epinephrine	—	1–4 μg/min	Alpha, beta agonist	Tachycardia, hypertension
Esmolol	500 μg/kg/min ×1 min	50–300 μg/kg/min	Beta blocker	Hypotension
Inamrinone	0.75 mg/kg over 2–3 mins	5–10 μg/kg/min	Phosphodiesterase inhibitor, inotrope	Hypotension, thrombocytopenia
Labetalol	20–40 mg q20min	0.5–2 mg/min	Alpha, beta blocker	Bronchospasm
Milrinone	50 μg/kg over 10 min	0.25–1 μg/kg/min	Phosphodiesterase inhibitor, inotrope	Hypotension, caution in renal impairment
Nitroglycerin	—	5–200 μg/min	Direct vasodilator	Headache
Nitroprusside	—	0.25–10 μg/kg/min	Direct vasodilator	Cyanide toxicity
Norepinephrine	—	2–10 μg/min	Alpha, beta agonist	Arrhythmias
Phenylephrine	—	10–100 μg/min	Alpha agonist	Reflex bradycardia

63

Bleeding

Emily R. Winslow

. . . all bleeding stops eventually . . .

You will encounter the bleeding patient in numerous situations throughout your time as a surgical house officer. The gunshot victim in the ER, the postoperative patient with a falling hematocrit, the woman with a saturated dressing in the recovery room, and the hypotensive man with bright red blood per rectum all will force you to deal with blood loss adeptly and rapidly.

DON'T PANIC

- The first and most important principle is *not to panic*. To most patients, the sight of blood is not a normal, everyday occurrence, and they often will begin to panic. You must not join the mass frenzy that often surrounds a bleeding patient. Instead, act deliberately and calmly to take care of the problem as rapidly as possible.

- Start by obtaining the patient's current vital signs and review the ABCs, as doing so will immediately tell you how serious the problem is.

- Remember that a young patient has greater physiologic reserves than does someone older. It takes greater blood loss to affect vital signs in the young.

VENOUS ACCESS

- Your first priority is to ensure you have a means for replacing the lost blood. Any patient with significant blood loss needs two large-bore (16 gauge) IV lines that function properly.

- If the patient does not have adequate peripheral veins for this, a central venous catheter should be placed. Use a Cordis catheter, not a typical triple-lumen catheter. See Appendix A, Procedures, for details about optimal placement sites.

RESUSCITATION

- In any circumstance in which a patient has lost a large volume of blood or the amount of blood loss is unclear, your next priority is to ensure that the patient receives aggressive and early volume resuscitation. This usually means immediately hooking up a liter of isotonic IV fluid on a pressure bag to a large-bore IV line.

- When the bleeding is ongoing and profuse, it may require immediate transfusion of packed RBCs.

- Familiarize yourself with how to obtain O negative blood from your hospital's blood bank for emergency release.

- Remember that postoperative patients often have crossmatched blood available in the blood bank.

HAVE BLOOD AVAILABLE

- Whenever you suspect that a patient may be bleeding, your damage control policy should be to ensure the patient has blood available in the blood bank.

- Call the blood bank to see if the patient has a type and screen, and find out when it expires. If the patient does not have a sample already, draw one to send immediately.

- Have the blood bank set up an adequate number of units for the problem at hand.

- Do not wait for CBC results or the patient to show signs of hemodynamic instability before setting up blood.

ETIOLOGY

- Sometimes the source is obvious, such as a spurting punctured dialysis access graft or a massive lower GI bleed.

- Always think of things that were recently done to the patient (e.g., cardiac catheterization, intraabdominal surgery, chest tube placement) and things that the patient is at risk for (e.g., delayed splenic rupture, stress gastritis, pulmonary hemorrhage).

- You may need to arrange immediate imaging studies (CT, angiogram, or nuclear studies) if appropriate and if the patient is stable for transport. Always consider the possibility that the early postoperative patient may need to return to the OR.

CONTRIBUTING FACTORS

The body's natural response to bleeding is clotting. If the patient has ongoing bleeding, the insult is so large that the body's ability to clot has been overwhelmed or the patient is not clotting properly. Things to check any time a patient is bleeding include

- PT and PTT

- Platelet count

- Body temperature: Hypothermic patients do not clot properly. Use warming blankets and heated IV fluid to increase core temperature.

- Medications: Stop any medications that could cause bleeding, including aspirin, warfarin (Coumadin), heparin, and ketorolac (Toradol). Stopping anticoagulants may be a difficult decision in circumstances in which the bleeding is not life threatening, but the consequences of stopping anticoagulation are. Consult your senior resident.

- Renal function: Uremic patients have impaired platelets. Consider DDAVP, as it will cause von Willlebrand's factor to be released and help initiate platelet aggregation.

COMPLICATIONS
Cardiac Function

Any patient with limited cardiac reserve (severe coronary artery disease, left ventricular dysfunction) is sensitive to impaired oxygen carrying capacity. Check an ECG to make sure there is no ongoing ischemia, and send the appropriate blood tests to rule out a silent myocardial infarction (troponin-I or CK-MB).

Pulmonary Function

Fear of volume overload is often cited as the reason for "gentle volume resuscitation" in the face of ongoing hemorrhage. Bleeding is a life-threatening complication, and if, in correcting it, you err on the side of volume overload and respiratory failure, the patient can be intubated and excess fluid removed with diuretics or dialysis. There is no excuse for underresuscitation.

Renal Function

Place a Foley catheter and monitor urine output.

AFTER THE INITIAL RESUSCITATION
Observing for Rebleeding

Observe the patient closely for rebleeding.

- Move the patient to a closely monitored setting.

- Check the vital signs frequently.

- Visit the patient frequently during the next several hours to assess the response to your interventions. If the patient is not following the expected trajectory, reassess the situation.

Checking the Hematocrit

We have intentionally listed this last on the list of priorities, although in practice it is often given first priority. Hematocrit can be very dangerous to rely on, because it is often the last value to change. Serial hematocrits can be useful, as they indicate the trend over a period of time.

VIII Nutrition

. . . if the gut works, use it . . .

Good nutrition is essential for timely recovery. Malnourished patients are at risk for infection, wound complications, and overall poorer outcome. Although not every surgical patient can be fed enterally, your patient's diet and nutrition status should always be on your mind.

Make frequent use of the dietitians at your institution. They can help craft custom meal plans for patients and also help you to estimate calorie needs and plan tube feedings or TPN.

64

Common Surgical Diets

Jeremy Goodman

REGULAR

- Standard hospital diet without specific restrictions.
- Is usually suitable for the surgical patient who is ready to eat solids and whose comorbidities do not require restrictions.

CLEAR LIQUID

- Clear juices (no citrus), thin broths, and Jello.
- Is completely absorbed in the small intestine.
- Postoperative patients are often begun on this diet after general anesthesia before advancing to more solid foods.
- Also suitable for the patient having a bowel prep.

FULL LIQUID

- Adds thicker liquids (citrus juice, milk, cream soups) to the diet.
- Sometimes used as a transition between clear liquids and a solid diet.

BLENDERIZED/PUREED

- Designed for patients after head, neck, or esophageal surgery and those with dysphagia who must avoid a solid food bolus.

SOFT

- Has fiber, texture, and seasoning modifications for patients unable to tolerate a regular diet.

POSTGASTRECTOMY

- Multiple small meals throughout the day are substituted for the traditional three large meals.
- Carbohydrates are limited to help prevent dumping syndrome.
- Beverages and liquids at meals are limited to help prevent early satiety.

FIBER RESTRICTED

- A low-residue diet designed to reduce feces and prevent blockage at strictures.
- Commonly used during intestinal inflammatory states.

HIGH FIBER

- There is some controversy over the effectiveness of this diet, but it has been variously recommended for the prevention of constipation, colon cancer, and diverticulitis.

LOW FAT

- Often given to patients with, or at high risk for, atherosclerotic disease.
- Also given to patients with fat malabsorption.

SODIUM RESTRICTED

- There are several types of diet that may be low in sodium.
- You may specify the amount of sodium in the diet (e.g., 2-g sodium diet).

DIABETIC

- In calorie-restricted diabetic diets, you may specify the number of calories (e.g., 1800-calorie diabetic diet). Non–calorie restricted is another option.
- The relative proportions of fats, carbohydrates, and proteins in these diets are monitored.

RENAL

- Modified in protein, phosphorus, potassium, sodium, and fluid content.
- Patient needs vary considerably depending on the type and efficiency of dialysis.

65

Estimating Nutritional Needs

Jeremy Goodman

CALORIES

Caloric needs can be determined in a number of ways. Remember that surgery and illness impose additional needs over the basal state.

- Simple estimate: 25–35 kcal/kg/day

- Harris-Benedict equation: basal energy expenditure

  - Men = 66.47 + [13.75 × weight (kg)] + [5 × height (cm)] – (6.76 × age)

  - Women = 655.1 + (9.56 × weight) + (1.85 × height) – (4.68 × age)

  - Stress factors: Multiply by basal
    - Minor operation: 1.2
    - Skeletal trauma: 1.35
    - Major sepsis: 1.6
    - Severe thermal injury: 2.1

- Estimate daily caloric requirements from carbohydrate and fat calories, not from proteins.

FAT

25–30% of total calories

PROTEIN

1–1.5 g/kg/day for maintenance; severely stressed patients may need as much as 2.5 g/kg/day.

66

Tube Feeding

Jeremy Goodman

For patients unable to take food by mouth, nutrition may be delivered through feeding tubes. A number of tube-feeding products exist, and names vary by brand. However, basic formulations are common across manufacturers.

- **Standard:** Generally 1 kcal/cc and suitable for most patients.

- **Volume-restricted:** 1.5–2 kcal/cc for patients who cannot tolerate excess volume. These solutions are hyperosmolar and may cause diarrhea.

- **Renal:** A low-volume, high-calorie, electrolyte-modified formulation for patients with acute or chronic renal failure.

- **High protein:** Ideal for those with high protein needs, such as burned or malnourished patients.

- **Pulmonary:** A low-carbohydrate, low–respiratory quotient formula that reduces CO_2 production when CO_2 retention is a concern.

- **Elemental:** Composed of simple sugars, amino acids, and lipids that require minimal digestion for complete absorption.

- **Immune enhancing:** Designed to reduce infections in the perioperative period, although their clinical value is questionable.

67 Total Parenteral Nutrition

Jeremy Goodman

- TPN is recommended for patients who require complete bowel rest for an extended period of time.

- Most people can tolerate bowel rest (with appropriate IV hydration) for approximately 7–10 days. Beyond that, significant malnutrition results. Therefore, consider TPN for any patient expected to require bowel rest for ≥7 days. It may also benefit malnourished preoperative patients who are unable to tolerate enteral feeding.

- Although significant advances have been made in TPN formulations, it is generally agreed that enteral feeding is healthier and more physiologic and should be used whenever possible.

- TPN must be delivered through a central vein because of its high osmolarity. Many institutions offer peripheral parenteral nutrition, which can be given via a peripheral vein. It is not as nutritionally complete as TPN, however, and is delivered in a larger volume of fluid.

- A patient on TPN needs routine measurement of electrolytes as well as liver function tests and triglycerides. Frequent blood glucose measurements should also be made, especially at the initiation of TPN. Insulin may be required in the feeding to help normalize blood sugars.

68

Nothing by Mouth (NPO)

Jeremy Goodman

- Remember that PO intake restriction is not a physiologic state. We often require our patients to fast for extended periods of time, whether in preparation for a procedure or for protection of abdominal structures.

- For periods of NPO longer than a few hours, IV fluid is essential to prevent dehydration and electrolyte abnormalities. A commonly used maintenance IV fluid is 5% dextrose in half normal saline with supplemental potassium (written as $D_5\frac{1}{2}NS$ with 20 mEq KCl/L). This solution is appropriate for the vast majority of patients who are unable to eat.

- Remember that prolonged NPO status should trigger a consideration of TPN.

69

Diabetes

Jeremy Goodman

- The diabetic patient presents a unique challenge from a dietary and glucose regulatory standpoint.

- Surgical diabetic patients should have their blood glucose levels assessed frequently by bedside fingerstick monitoring. A blood glucose level <200 mg/dL should be your target, as higher glucose levels impair wound healing and alter the immune response.

HYPOGLYCEMIC MEDICATIONS

- Although some diabetics are able to regulate their blood glucose through diet and exercise alone, the majority of your patients will be taking some kind of hypoglycemic agent. These include PO agents and/or insulin.

- As a general rule, most patients can be left off their PO agents temporarily and hyperglycemia treated with intermittent subcutaneous insulin.

- Do not give fasting patients PO hypoglycemics. For insulin-dependent diabetics, give half their normal dose of insulin when fasting.

- Remember that type I, or juvenile, diabetics produce no insulin and always must be given some supplemental insulin.

SLIDING SCALE

Even non–insulin-dependent diabetics will benefit from a "sliding-scale" insulin regimen. Infection, surgery, and stress have a negative impact on glycemic control, and the patient's outpatient medication regimen may not be sufficient. A sliding-scale insulin order provides varying insulin dosages based on blood glucose ranges. Perform fingerstick monitoring q4–6h, and give subcutaneous regular insulin no more frequently than that. A sample sliding scale is illustrated below:

BLOOD GLUCOSE	ORDER
<60	Give juice (if conscious and not NPO) or IV dextrose ($\frac{1}{2}$–1 ampule D_{50}) and call M.D.
61–150	No insulin
151–200	2 U regular insulin SC
201–250	4 U regular insulin SC
251–300	6 U regular insulin SC
301–350	8 U regular insulin SC
>351	10 U regular insulin SC and call M.D.

Check daily to see how much sliding-scale insulin the patient has required. Increase the standing insulin order if >8–10 U of sliding-scale insulin were given on the previous day.

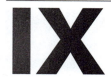 # Tubes and Drains

. . . a tube in every orifice . . .

Nearly every surgical inpatient will, at some time, have a tube or drain placed. Although specific indications for each piece of equipment vary, tubes and drains accomplish two basic goals: introduction of needed substances and evacuation of undesirable ones. We consider the most common types found in the surgical patient.

70

Nasoenteric Tubes

Jeremy Goodman

NASOGASTRIC TUBES

- NG tubes serve the dual purposes of evacuation and introduction.

- They can be placed to acutely decompress the stomach and can be left in for an extended period of time to provide continuous drainage in the setting of a gastric or bowel obstruction.

- They also prevent swallowed air from accumulating in the patient with a bowel obstruction.

- In the patient who is not able to swallow food or medications by mouth, NG tubes provide a convenient route for administration.

- NG tubes should *not* be placed in the patient with massive facial trauma or in whom you suspect basilar skull fracture. In these settings, consider an orogastric tube.

- See Appendix A for details on NG tube placement.

NASODUODENAL TUBES

- Nasoduodenal tubes are small-caliber (usually 10 or 12 French), 40- to 50-in. long tubes used when there is concern that gastric feeding may lead to aspiration.

- Note that due to the small lumen of these tubes, crushed medications should *not* be given through them.

- See Appendix A for details on placement of nasoduodenal tubes.

71

Surgically Placed Feeding Tubes

Jeremy Goodman

Surgically placed feeding tubes include gastrostomy tubes (G-tubes) and jejunostomy tubes (J-tubes). These are almost exclusively used for introduction of enteral feedings and medication, although gastrostomy tubes may occasionally be used for gastric drainage. A jejunostomy tube is preferred when the risk for aspiration exists, as feedings are introduced distal to the pylorus.

GASTROSTOMY TUBES

- Gastrostomy tubes may be placed through an open or percutaneous route. The *open* procedure is performed in the OR and involves making a small upper abdominal incision, identifying the stomach, inserting the tube, and suturing it in place. The stomach is often sutured up to the abdominal wall to reduce the risk of leak, and the incision is closed. These tubes should generally be left to gravity drainage for 24–48 hrs before use.

- The *percutaneous* procedure may be performed at the ICU bedside, endoscopy suite, or OR. An endoscope is passed through the mouth into the stomach, and a needle is introduced through the abdominal wall under direct scope visualization. Once the needle has passed into the stomach, a wire is passed and withdrawn through the mouth. The feeding tube, or PEG (percutaneous endoscopic gastrostomy), is then advanced over the wire in the manner of a modified Seldinger technique and pulled through the abdominal wall. A retaining clip is attached to the tube, and it is sutured to the abdominal skin. These tubes should generally be left to gravity drainage for 48 hrs before use.

JEJUNOSTOMY TUBES

- Jejunostomy tubes are almost always placed by the open technique, although there are percutaneous and laparoscopic methods. In the open procedure, the jejunum is identified, and a tube is placed into the lumen. The exterior of the jejunum may be sutured over the tube to create a tunnel, or it may be sutured to the abdominal wall, similar to the gastrostomy tube. These tubes generally do not need to be left to gravity drainage initially and are almost exclusively used for feeding.

GENERAL CONSIDERATIONS

- Feeding tubes can clog easily, and you will be called when the nurses cannot unclog them. There are several strategies for unclogging feeding tubes. Forceful injection of water or saline will usually have been tried before your arrival but should be repeated. To dissolve a blockage, several products, such as cola, meat tenderizer, or pancreatic enzyme capsules dissolved in water, can be instilled into the tube. As a last resort, tubes that have been indwelling for several weeks can sometimes be replaced at the bedside.

- You can also attempt to replace a tube that has fallen out. Before replacing a tube, know the technique used to place it initially. It is generally not possible to replace a tunneled gastrostomy or jejunostomy tube once it has fallen out. **Check with a senior resident before attempting to replace.**

  - Before using a replaced tube, confirm correct position and that there is no leak by injecting a small amount of water-soluble contrast and taking an x-ray.

72 Tracheostomy

Jeremy Goodman

A tracheostomy may be placed permanently, in the setting of neck surgery, or temporarily, to facilitate weaning from mechanical ventilation.

- It is placed inferior to the vocal cords, and patients with functioning tracheostomies cannot talk without a special valve. Many, however, can eat with a tracheostomy in place.

- Tracheostomy tubes come in many varieties, with differences in diameter, composition of tube and cuff, fenestration, and length.

- If the tracheostomy tube becomes dislodged, immediately try to replace it. If the patient is ventilator dependent, and the tube cannot be easily and immediately replaced, endotracheally intubate the patient. Make sure to position the endotracheal tube cuff inferior to the tracheostomy stoma. Tracheostomy tube replacement can then be undertaken in a more controlled fashion.

- Bleeding from a new tracheostomy is not uncommon and is usually self-limited in the patient without coagulopathy. For persistent bleeding, a small amount of Surgicel or Gelfoam can be placed over the bleeding areas.

- A rare bleeding consequence of tracheostomy is erosion into the innominate artery, leading to profound bleeding. As the artery lies superficial to the trachea, you may place a finger into the stoma and compress the artery between the trachea and the chest wall until help arrives.

- **Notify your senior resident of any bleeding immediately.**

73

Closed Suction Drain

Jeremy Goodman

Drains are placed intraoperatively when there is concern for anticipated bleeding, leak, or infection. They provide a mechanism for continuous evacuation of a specific area, as well as for visualization and testing of draining fluid.

- Bulb suction drains are attached to a plastic or rubber reservoir (often called a grenade), which is squeezed empty. The vacuum generated by this provides for continuous suction. The two most common drains attached to such a reservoir are Jackson-Pratt and Blake drains. Jackson-Pratt drains are flat with multiple holes, and Blake drains are cylindric with long channels. Both can be removed at the bedside by releasing the suction from the reservoir, removing the anchoring suture, and pulling steadily until the drain comes out. Inspect the end of the drain to make sure it does not look ragged, which would suggest that it has broken off during removal.

- Bulb suction drains should be "stripped" periodically. Starting closest to the insertion site, pinch the external tubing between your thumb and forefinger and use your other hand to milk the tubing down to the bulb. This action pulls clot out of the tubing and into the reservoir. Make sure to hold the drain in place at the skin with your other hand to prevent dislodging it.

- Davall, or sump, drains are large-caliber, triple-lumen tubes that can be used for continuous irrigation and suction of the abdominal cavity.

- Hemovac collection chambers are large cylinders with a spring in the middle. After the air in the chamber is evacuated and the spring compressed, slow expansion of the spring provides continuous suction.

X

Surgical Subspecialties: Neurosurgery

Recognizing that many surgical interns and medical students rotate through surgical subspecialty services (and there is coverage of subspecialty material in standardized exams), efforts were undertaken to include the same type of practical advice from those in neurosurgery, orthopedic surgery, urology, and plastic surgery. The following sections were written independently, but they are intended to be complementary to the material in the *Surgery Survival Guide*. Although brief, each reflects what the authors feel are key points to remember when approaching patients in that particular subspecialty. We hope you will find them a useful addition.

Tammy L. Lin, M.D.
Series Editor

74 Neurosurgery Essentials

Eric C. Leuthardt and Douglas John Fox, Jr.

NEUROLOGIC EXAM

- The neurosurgical patient can have a very dynamic, rapidly changing exam.

- In caring for a neurosurgical patient, one always should be up to date regarding current neurologic status.

- The basic components of the exam are as follows and should be presented in this order:

  - Glasgow Coma Scale

  - Level of consciousness: awake, somnolent, lethargic, obtunded, comatose

  - Cranial nerves: pupils (are they reactive?), extraocular muscles, face, tongue midline (TML)

  - Motor: drift on Barre? Strength in all extremities (0–5 scale)

- Any time there is a change in neurologic status, notify the neurosurgical house officer.

HEAD CT

- If there is any question about a change in a patient's neurologic status, you will never be faulted for getting a head CT. A head CT to the neurosurgeon is a fundamental diagnostic tool and is the same as a chest x-ray to the cardiothoracic surgeon, an ECG to the cardiologist, or a KUB to the general surgeon. A head CT is a fundamental diagnostic tool.

- Head CTs are vital in assessing *mass effect* of intracranial lesions, are very sensitive for intracranial hemorrhage (subdural, epidural, and subarachnoid), and allow one to assess the size of the ventricles (i.e., hydrocephalus).

MOST COMMONLY USED MEDICATIONS

- Phenytoin (PHT, Dilantin):

  - Loading: 18 mg/kg IV (usually 1 g for average patient)

  - Maintenance: 300 mg PO qhs

- Dexamethasone (Decadron): 4 mg IV/PO q6h
- Nimodipine (Nimotop): 60 mg PO q4h
- Mannitol (Osmitrol, Resectisol):
  - Emergent: 100 g IV ×1
  - Maintenance: 50 g IV q4h

75

Neurosurgery: General Approach

Eric C. Leuthardt and Douglas John Fox, Jr.

"COMMUNICATION, COMMUNICATION, AND COMMUNICATION . . ."

Neurosurgeons deal with a broad spectrum of illnesses involving the brain and spinal cord. As an intern on a neurosurgical service, you are responsible for first-line evaluation of floor and possibly ICU and consult patients. As with any high-acuity service, *communication is essential*. If there are problems with a patient, they must be addressed quickly, with the problem identified proactively and senior neurosurgical staff notified soon after. The common types of neurosurgical patients include

- Trauma (intracranial and spinal)

- Subarachnoid hemorrhage (often secondary to aneurysmal rupture)

- Brain and spinal tumors

- Patients with spinal degenerative disease

You are an important member of the neurosurgical team, and your role as a part of that team is to act as the first line in assessment and management of your patients.

CLINICAL EVALUATION: "THE SAME WAY EVERY TIME" AND "ASYMMETRY IS THE NAME OF THE GAME"
Initial Evaluation

In the initial assessment of any neurosurgical patient, the primary survey should always be included. Namely, the ABCs, as well as a basic cardiovascular (including evaluation for carotid bruits and distal pulses), pulmonary, and abdominal exam.

The neurologic exam among neurosurgical residents has been standardized so that it serves for easy communication and assessment of a clinical situation. The essential component of the exam is to assess for any asymmetry, which may indicate a localizable neurosurgical problem. The format is as follows:

- **Glasgow Coma Scale:** think of it as the fundamental vital signs for a neurosurgery patient (Table 75-1):

TABLE 75-1.
GLASGOW COMA SCALE

Components	Points
Eye opening	
Spontaneous	4
To voice	3
To stimulation	2
None	1
Motor response	
To command	6
Localizes	5
Withdraws	4
Abnormal flexion	3
Extension	2
None	1
Verbal response	
Oriented	5
Confused but comprehensible	4
Incoherent	3
Incomprehensible (no words)	2
None	1

- **Mental status:**
  - Level of consciousness: Several basic levels of consciousness include
    - *Awake*: eyes open and talking
    - *Somnolent*: eyes closed, but open to voice
    - *Lethargic*: eyes closed, but open to pain
    - *Obtunded*: eyes closed, do not open to voice or painful stimuli (To say that a patient is sleepy is not adequate.)
  - Orientation: Does the patient know the following 3 things?
    - Name
    - The place patient is located (i.e., name of the hospital)
    - Year and date

If yes, the patient is "oriented to person, place, and time"; if no, the patient is "*confused*, and oriented to (whatever the patient answered correctly)."

- Speech:
  - Does the patient look at you or *regard*? Does the patient follow commands and speak normally? If yes, the patient "*regards, follows commands*, and has *clear and fluent speech*."
  - If not, does the patient not regard? Does the patient not follow commands? Does the patient not understand what you are saying (*receptive aphasia*), or can the patient understand but not produce coherent speech (*expressive aphasia*)?
  - Note: a lethargic neurosurgical patient has increased ICP until proved otherwise!

- **Cranial nerve (CN) exam:**
  - Pupils (CNs II and III): Assess pupils' size and reactivity to light—are they *brisk, sluggish*, or *nonreactive*?
  - Extraocular movements (CNs III, IV, and VI): Assess that eyes move in all directions.
    - Third nerve palsy: Patient's eye is deviated laterally with a dilated, nonreactive pupil. A third nerve palsy is an indicator of herniation due to elevated ICP or a mass lesion and should be considered an emergent situation.
  - Face (CN VII):
    - Is the smile symmetric, and does the patient raise his or her eyebrows equally?
    - Is the facial weakness *central* (smile asymmetry only) or *peripheral* (smile and eyebrow asymmetry)?
  - Facial sensation (CN V): Is sensation to light touch and pinprick the same on both sides?
  - Hearing (CN VIII): Can the patient hear equally on both sides as you rub your fingers together?
  - Tongue (CN XII): Is the patient's tongue midline? It deviates to the side of the palsy.

- **Motor exam:**
  - *Barre test*: A *very sensitive* exam for cortical dysfunction.
    - Method: Have the patient hold arms in front of him or her with palms supinated—"Hold your arms out like you're holding a pizza."

- Results: If a patient begins to pronate one hand and/or drop an arm, it represents a degree of cortical dysfunction on the contralateral hemisphere. This is reported as a *pronator drift on Barre*—know this exam.

- Motor testing: Assess strength in the following muscle groups:

  - deltoid
  - biceps
  - triceps
  - grip
  - intrinsic hand muscles
  - iliopsoas
  - quadriceps
  - hamstring
  - anterior tibialis (ankle dorsiflexion)
  - gastrocnemius (plantar flexion)
  - extensor hallucis longus (great toe extension)

  Grading scale: 5 = full strength; 4+ = slightly diminished strength with resistance; 4 = can overcome muscle with resistance; 4– = antigravity, can easily overcome muscle with resistance; 3 = can move muscle with gravity only; 2 = can move muscle, but not against gravity; 1 = twitches muscle; 0 = no movement.

- **Sensory exam:**

  - Assess fine touch, pinprick, joint position in all extremities.

  - In trauma patient, evaluate for *sensory level* (with pinprick): important landmarks for sensory dermatomes: T4: nipples; T10: umbilicus.

- **Reflexes:**

  - *Deep tendon reflexes*: The important ones include biceps (C5), supinator (C6), triceps (C7), knee (L3–4), and ankle (S1).

  - Grading of reflexes: 0 = none, 1 = trace, 2 = normal, 3 = hyperreflexic, 4 = clonus.

  - Pathologic reflexes: Primitive reflexes that are normally inhibited until there is some type of compromise to the corticospinal tract, or upper motor neuron lesion, that leads to their being released.

    - *Babinski* ("toes"): Scratching the bottom of the foot should cause the toes to curl downward (*toes are downgoing*). A positive Babinski or abnormal response is when, on scratching the sole of the foot, the toes point upward (toward the head; *toes are upgoing*).

- *Hoffmann's*: A pathologic response is elicited by snapping the distal phalanx of the middle finger, which causes the thumb to flex.

- **Cerebellar exam:**

  - *Finger to nose*: Have the patient touch his or her nose and then your finger, which should be approximately 3 ft in front of the patient. If the patient misses or goes beyond your finger, there is *upper extremity dysmetria*.

  - *Heel to shin*: Have the patient run his or her heel on the opposite shin. If the patient is clumsy or is unable to, there is *lower extremity dysmetria*.

- **Gait and station:** If possible, have the patient stand and walk approximately 10 ft. Assess whether the patient has any *postural instability* (i.e., is the patient able to stand up straight without falling to one side or the other?), or gait difficulties/unsteadiness (i.e., is the gait *wide based* or *shuffling*, or does the patient fall to one side more than the other?).

DOCUMENTING A NORMAL EXAM

MS: AAO × 3, regards, FC, speech C & F
CN: PERL 3/3 – 2/2. EOMI, FACE =, V123 = LT, TML
MOTOR: Without drift on Barre

	DELT	B	TRII	GRIP	INT	IP	QUAD	HAM	GAST	AT	EHL
Right	5	5	5	5	5	5	5	5	5	5	5
Left	5	5	5	5	5	5	5	5	5	5	5

Sensory: intact to LT/PP/JP (light touch, pinprick, joint position), without sensory level

Reflexes:

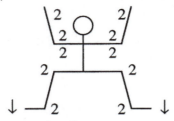

Negative Hoffmann's
Nl cerebellar exam
Nl gait and station

76 Approach to Common Problems in Neurosurgery

Eric C. Leuthardt and Douglas John Fox, Jr.

MENTAL STATUS CHANGES

First one must decide how the patient is different:

- Has the level of consciousness changed?
- Is the patient more confused?
- Is the patient agitated?

When there is a mental status change, one must perform a full neurologic exam with vital signs.

Many processes can cause an altered level of consciousness, confusion, and agitation. The neurosurgeon's job is to make sure that the change is not related to a life-threatening increase in ICP.

The exam may allow a more tailored approach, but in general you should evaluate the following items:

- Vital signs: oxygenation, heart rate, BP, temp
- Neurologic exam: look for changes from the baseline
- Medications (i.e., narcotics, sedatives, steroids)
- Medical history and basic heart, lung, and abdominal exam
- Lab analysis, including electrolytes, arterial oxygen saturation, ECG, CBC, and UA/microscopy

For the neurosurgical patient, perform a head CT scan if there is any concern for the patient's status being related to increased ICP. Remember that as long as the patient is stable, a head CT can only help in your determination of the problem at hand. Having a normal head CT in a deteriorating patient shows that there is not a neurosurgical lesion to be addressed.

When a patient's exam changes, start the workup and let the senior house staff know to ensure that the patient is worked up adequately.

HYPONATREMIA

Hyponatremia is a common problem on the neurosurgical service; the most important electrolyte to brain function is sodium.

Hyponatremia is a condition that may occur with fluid overload, as in congestive heart failure, but in the neurosurgical patient one must consider the SIADH and cerebral salt wasting (CSW). Hyponatremia is not well tolerated by the CNS in general, but sudden shifts in the sodium level can cause similar problems, even when the total drop in the serum sodium is not as severe.

Cerebral Salt Wasting

- Occurs when the kidneys lose water and sodium as a result of intracranial pathology (i.e., subarachnoid hemorrhage).

- Patients have decreased plasma volume, negative salt balance, and signs and symptoms of dehydration.

- Serum potassium may be increased, a finding that is incompatible with SIADH.

- May be difficult to differentiate from SIADH, but two important differences are extracellular volume and total body salt balance; wedge and central venous pressure will be low in CSW.

- Treated with fluid resuscitation and sodium replacement.

- May exacerbate vasospasm secondary to negative fluid balance.

SIADH

- Is diagnosed when the serum sodium is diluted with a normal or increased intravascular volume.

- Occurs with the release of antidiuretic hormone without osmotic stimuli and results in dilutional hyponatremia with high urine osmolality.

- Etiologies include meningitis, brain tumors (e.g., pituitary), head trauma, increased ICP, malignant tumors (e.g., bronchogenic lung cancer), drug-induced causes (e.g., thiazide diuretics).

- Diagnostic criteria include hyponatremia, low serum sodium and concentrated urine, and normal renal function.

- Symptoms include nausea, emesis, lethargy, confusion, and seizures.

- Treatment is fluid restriction with close following of the serum sodium unless severe, which may require hypertonic saline and medications [e.g., furosemide (Lasix), demeclocycline (Declomycin), phenytoin (Dilantin)].

- Correction must be done slowly to limit the risk of central pontine myelinolysis, in which osmotic changes cause demyelination of the pontine and other white matter tracts, resulting in mental status changes, flaccid quadriplegia, and cranial nerve changes.

HYPERNATREMIA
Diabetes Insipidus

Diabetes insipidus (DI) is a common cause of hypernatremia in neurosurgery patients. DI is frequently encountered in the following types of patients:

- Patient's status post–transphenoidal surgery for sellar and suprasellar masses, such as pituitary adenomas and craniopharyngiomas

- Severe traumatic head injury

Patients in DI must fulfill the following three criteria:

- Na >146

- Urine specific gravity <1.005

- Urine output >250 cc/hr for ≥2 hrs

When a patient fulfills these three criteria, there are several management steps:

- Initial management:

  - Allow the patient to drink as dictated by thirst.

  - Have a pitcher of water placed at bedside.

  - Follow intake and output closely.

  - Repeat serum Na in 4–6 hrs.

- If conservative measures fail:

  - If patient becomes progressively more volume depleted (i.e., patient is unable to match output with PO fluid input), attempt to match urine output with IV hydration using $D_5\frac{1}{2}$ normal saline replacing 2/3 cc/cc of urine output.

- If patient continues to outpace IV fluid hydration (urine output >300 cc ×4 hrs or 500–800 cc/hr):

  - Give desmopressin DDAVP: 2.5–5 µg SC ×1.

  - Repeat Na in 4–6 hrs.

SEIZURES

In the neurosurgical patient, a seizure may occur for the following common reasons:

- Neurologic insult: after trauma (closed head injury or penetrating head injury), CNS infection (meningitis, abscess, empyema), fevers/sepsis, or stroke

- CNS anatomic abnormality: Brain tumor, arteriovenous malformation, or other mass lesions (subdural hematoma, epidural hematoma)

- Metabolic disturbances:
  - Electrolyte disturbances: most notably *hyponatremia*, hypocalcemia, and profound hypoglycemia
- Alcohol withdrawal
- Other drugs: cocaine, Demerol, Darvon, PCP

Initial Evaluation

Important elements of history:

- Was this seizure witnessed? Did the patient localize (i.e., did it start in one location, suggesting an anatomic correlation)?
- Does this patient have a drug or alcohol history?
- Any fevers?
- Is this patient already on anticonvulsants?

Physical Exam

Important aspects of physical exam:

- Start with the ABCs: Make sure the patient has an airway and is able to protect it, is breathing, and has adequate oxygen saturation and stable hemodynamics.
- Mental status: Is patient lethargic, confused (= *postictal*)?
- Cranial nerve/motor exam: Is there anything different in the patient's exam from before his or her seizure (e.g., new cranial nerve deficits or new motor weakness after the seizure, otherwise known as *Todd's paralysis*)?
- Does the patient have signs of meningeal infection [neck stiffness (*nuchal rigidity*), sensitivity to light (*photophobia*)]?

Diagnostic Evaluation

- Anatomic etiology: **Head CT:** rule out any acute surgically correctable or anatomic source for the seizures (enlarging contusion, subdural hematoma, epidural hematoma, brain tumor, arteriovenous malformation, or stroke).
- Metabolic etiology: Blood glucose, serum electrolytes (including calcium and magnesium), CBC, and ABG; if the patient is already on an anticonvulsant (e.g., phenytoin), check a serum level.
- Lumbar puncture: If there is concern for infection without an identified source (e.g., negative UA, chest x-ray), rule out meningitis. **Do not perform lumbar puncture until a mass lesion has been ruled out with a head CT.**

Treatment

- Correct any metabolic abnormality or hypoxia.

- *Status epilepticus (SE) is a medical emergency.*

  - SE is defined as seizures >30 mins, but aggressive measures to "break" the seizure activity should be undertaken if the seizures persist >10 mins.

  - Goals in SE are to stabilize the patient, stop the seizure, and identify the etiology.

  - Initial management: ABCs (as above), gain IV access (two lines are preferable).

  - Standard protocol for SE in adults:

    1. Lorazepam (Ativan), 4 mg IV slowly over 2 mins; repeat in 5 mins if seizures persist.
    2. Simultaneously load with phenytoin: 1200 mg IV if not on phenytoin, 500 mg if already on phenytoin.
    3. If seizures persist: Phenobarbital (20 mg/kg, max. 1400 mg) infused at approximately 100 mg/min until seizure stops. (*Watch out for hypotension!*)
    4. If seizures persist >30 mins, intubate (if not done already) and begin general anesthesia. Most commonly used: load—pentobarbital 15 mg/kg at 25 mg/min; maintenance—2.5 mg/kg/hr until EEG burst suppression achieved.

BRAIN TUMORS

In broad terms, of the many types of brain tumors, there are those that are *metastatic* (arising from outside the cranial cavity) and those that are *primary* (tumors derived from the brain or its associated structures).

The most common *metastatic* tumors (in decreasing order of incidence) are:

- Lung cancer

- Breast cancer

- Renal cell cancer

- Melanoma

The most common *primary* tumors are

- Astrocytomas—glioblastoma multiforme

- Anaplastic astrocytoma

- Low-grade astrocytoma

- Meningioma

- Pituitary adenomas

Evaluation

Clinical Aspects

How a patient will present is extremely variable depending on the location, size, and type of tumor. Common complaints are headache, progressive motor weakness, and seizures.

Important Aspects of the History

- Duration of symptoms?
- How rapidly have the symptoms progressed?
- Any history of cancer?
- Does the patient smoke or drink?
- Do any tumors or cancers run in the family?

Important Aspects of the Physical Exam

- Mental status
- Vision field deficit?
- Double vision?
- Third nerve palsy?
- Motor weakness?
  - The lethargic patient has mass effect from the tumor until proven otherwise—this is an emergency!
- Tests:
  - Labs include all preop labs: CBC, electrolyte panel, PT/PTT, type and screen, UA
  - Imaging:
    - Head CT (if not already done) to quickly rule out mass effect
    - Metastatic workup: Chest, abdominal, pelvic CTs; breast mammogram.
    - Tumor protocol: MRI (includes T1, T2, and T1 with contrast and diffusion-weighted imaging)—gold standard for evaluating tumor, brain anatomy, and mass effect of the lesion.
  - Questions to ask yourself or the radiologist reading the film:
    - Is the lesion intraaxial (in the brain) or extraaxial (outside the brain)?
    - Is there mass effect?
    - Is there midline shift, and if so, how much?

- Is there hydrocephalus?

- Is there significant edema?

- Is there one or multiple lesions?

- Treatment: Therapies are variable depending on the type and location of the tumor. They range from surgical resection, to biopsy, to radiation and chemotherapy. Initial management of an intracranial lesion involves controlling mass effect, if present, and providing prophylaxis against possible seizures.

- **Management of mass effect:**

  - Brain tumors are often associated with significant edema due to cytokine-induced capillary permeability; it can be stabilized with steroids.

    - Dexamethasone (Decadron), 10 mg IV bolus ×1 and maintenance of 4 mg IV/PO q4h

    - To prevent steroid-induced ulcers, all patients should be on gastric prophylaxis: famotidine (Pepcid), 20 mg IV/PO bid.

- **Seizure prophylaxis:**

  - Phenytoin: load—18 mg/kg IV (approximately 1 g); maintenance—300 mg PO qhs, 100 mg IV q8h, or 200 mg/tube bid

- Special note on pituitary adenomas:

  - These are often slow-growing tumors arising from the anterior aspect of the pituitary gland. They are divided into two categories: *functional* adenomas, which secrete various pituitary hormones (prolactin, growth hormone, and ACTH most commonly), and *nonfunctional*, which are endocrine inactive.

  - They often present with visual changes due to either the tumor's pressure on the chiasm (*bitemporal hemianopsia*, i.e., bilateral lateral field cuts) or a derangement of endocrine hyperfunction or hypofunction (menstrual/fertility irregularities, acromegaly, or Cushing's disease).

  - Primary evaluation of these tumors involves the following:

    - Endocrine evaluation: a.m. cortisol level, T_4/TSH, prolactin, FSH/estrogen/testosterone, insulin-like growth factor-1.

    - Visual function: formal visual field exam by ophthalmology

    - Anatomic evaluation: MRI with and without gadolinium contrast

HYDROCEPHALUS AND SHUNTS
Cerebrospinal Fluid

- The brain makes approximately 500 cc of CSF/day, or 20 cc/hr.

- CSF is created by the choroid plexus in the lateral ventricles. It passes through the foramen of Monroe to the third ventricle, after which it flows through the aqueduct of Sylvius to the fourth ventricle. The fluid then exits the fourth ventricle through the foramen of Magendie and Luschka to the basal cisterns and passes into the subarachnoid space, where it is eventually absorbed by the arachnoid granulations at the sagittal sinus.

- The interruption in the egress of CSF, which results in the enlargement of the ventricles and potentially an increase in ICP, is known as *hydrocephalus* (HCP).

Hydrocephalus

Two functional divisions of HCP:

- **Obstructive:** The mechanical blockage of CSF flow, often caused by tumors, congenital malformations (Chiari and Dandy Walker malformations), and large intraventricular hemorrhage.

- **Communicating:** Impairment of CSF absorption at the arachnoid granulations, often caused by meningitis and subarachnoid hemorrhage.

Acute HCP is a life-threatening emergency and must be addressed immediately.

Evaluation
Clinical
Acute HCP presents with symptoms of increasing ICP, which include headache, nausea/vomiting, lethargy, upgaze or sixth nerve palsies, gait problems, and papilledema.

Imaging
Head CT is the imaging modality of choice for assessment of HCP. Important aspects of head CT include the size of the ventricles (are they enlarged? larger than ventricles on previous CTs?) and whether the sulci are effaced.

Treatment
A patient with acute HCP requires emergent diversion of CSF to relieve elevated ICP. Two methods are available:

Ventriculostomy (Temporary)
A ventriculostomy is a catheter that is passed from the frontal horn of the lateral ventricle and tunneled under the skin; it exits to an externally

draining bag. The rate of external ventricular drainage, or the pressure against which CSF is allowed to egress, is controlled by the height of the drainage chamber relative to the tragus of the ear. The higher the chamber, the higher the pressure in the ventricle must be to overcome the resistance to CSF outflow. Usual starting chamber height is 10–15 cm above the tragus.

Shunt (Permanent)

A shunt is a permanent system that provides an alternate conduit of CSF drainage. It drains CSF from the ventricle into either the peritoneal cavity (*ventriculoperitoneal shunt*) or the atrium (*ventriculoatrial shunt*). Shunts are usually placed after patients are unable to wean off a ventriculostomy. Shunts are fallible constructs and can occasionally occlude or become infected.

Shunt malfunction may present in a variety of ways, ranging from symptoms of acute hydrocephalus due to occlusion, to meningitis due to infection of the shunt (fevers, neck stiffness, photophobia), to milder diffuse symptoms of chronic headache, nausea, and other vague complaints. Workup usually includes

- Head CT: Compare current head CT to prior CT to assess whether ventricular size is different.

- Shunt series (posteroanterior and lateral plain films of head, neck, chest, and abdomen) to assess whether areas of disconnection or kinking of the tubing apparatus exist.

- Possibly shunt tap for CSF, if infection suspected.

- Shuntogram: A radionuclide study in which a radioisotope (technetium) is injected into the reservoir of the shunt valve and followed with a gamma camera to assess flow of the isotope from the valve to the site of CSF diversion (e.g., the abdomen for ventriculoperitoneal shunts, and the atrium for ventriculoatrial shunts).

TRAUMA

Head trauma is a common situation on the neurosurgical service.

Closed Head Injury

Closed head injury refers to injury to the brain or its associated structure secondary to a large concussive force. Brain injury from trauma is the result of two distinct causes, primary and secondary injury.

Primary Injury

A primary injury is a direct result of impact damage and includes brain contusions, diffuse axonal injury, lacerations, and skull fractures.

Brain Contusion

A brain contusion is a primary brain lesion often related to sudden deceleration injury in which brain impacts against bone (i.e., temporal lobes, frontal lobes, and occipital lobes). It is usually characterized by intraparenchymal, heterogeneous high-density lesions. Surgical decompression may be required if herniation is imminent.

Diffuse Axonal Injury

A diffuse axonal injury is a primary lesion of rotational acceleration/deceleration that results in the diffuse microscopic shearing of axons. Evidence of this type of injury can occasionally be seen as small punctate hemorrhages in white matter regions, most notably in the corpus callosum and brain stem. These patients are often rendered comatose immediately after their injuries. This is a nonsurgical injury.

Secondary Injury

A secondary injury occurs subsequent to the impact; it includes hematomas, edema, hypoxia, and ischemia.

Intracranial Hemorrhages

- **Subdural hematoma (SDH):** Acute SDHs are usually due to the accumulation of blood around a brain laceration or a torn bridging surface vessel. On head CT, they appear as a crescent-shaped mass along the inner table of the skull. In general, if the patient is symptomatic and the SDH is >1 cm thick, *the lesion requires surgical evacuation emergently.*

- **Epidural hematoma (EDH):** Classically, EDHs are the result of a temporoparietal skull fracture that tears the middle meningeal artery, causing bleeding that dissects the dura away from the skull. These lesions occasionally present with a *lucid interval*, in which the patient has an initial posttraumatic loss of consciousness followed by a period of regained consciousness and then a subsequent neurologic decline. Head CT reveals a high-density biconvex-shaped lesion against the skull. If the patient is symptomatic, and/or the EDH is >1 cm, *the patient requires immediate surgical evacuation.*

Clinical Evaluation

General Exam

Important aspects of the history include any periods of *hypoxia, hypotension, seizures*, or *extensor/flexor posturing.*

Evaluate the usual ABCs with emphasis on the following special points:

- Look for evidence of basal skull fracture: *raccoon's eyes* (periorbital ecchymoses), *Battle's sign* (postauricular ecchymoses), CSF rhinorrhea/otorrhea, hemotympanum.

- Check for facial fractures.

- Auscultate over carotids for bruits to assess for possible dissection.

Neurologic Exam

- Glasgow Coma Scale (GCS): Severity of head injury is graded according to the GCS score (see Chap. 75, Neurosurgery: General Approach). Mild head injuries are 14–15, moderate 9–13, and severe ≤8.

- Cranial nerves (CN):

  - Pupils/CN III: Are the pupils reactive?

  - Extraocular movement: If the patient is not conscious, one may need to check *oculovestibular reflex* via *cold calorics*. In a comatose patient, injecting cold water into the ear canal should induce the eyes to deviate toward the side of injection (do not give the "doll's eye test" to a patient who has not had his or her cervical spine cleared.)

  - CN VII function: Can the patient raise his or her brow symmetrically? If not, the patient may have a temporal bone fracture affecting the peripheral seventh nerve.

- Motor: Is the patient moving all extremities? If comatose, does the patient move them to noxious stimuli? Is there rectal tone?

- Sensory: Is there a sensory level (if patient is cooperative enough to check)?

- Reflexes: Any evidence of increased tone—Babinski and Hoffmann's signs?

- Clinical signs of increased ICP (emergent situation requiring immediate intervention):

  - Progressive deterioration of neurologic status

  - Unilateral or bilateral pupillary dilation

  - Asymmetric pupillary reaction to light

  - Decerebrate or decorticate posturing

Lab Evaluation

- PT/PTT/INR (Patients with severe head injury are frequently coagulopathic and require transfusions of FFP/platelets.)

- CBC

- Electrolyte panel

- Type and screen

- **Head CT (ASAP)**

- Spine series: see Spinal Cord Injuries for more detail.

Management

Minor Head Injury (GCS 14–15)

- Admit to floor.

- Elevate head of bed to 30 degrees.

- Perform neurologic checks q2h.

- NPO.

- Acetaminophen for pain and antiemetics prn.

- IV fluids: D_5NS with 20 mEq KCl at 70–100 cc/hr

Moderate Head Injury (GCS 9–13)

- Admit to ICU.

- Same orders as above, with repeat head CT in a.m.

Severe Head Injury (GCS ≤8)

- **Intubation:** If demonstrating signs of increased ICP (as above), if GCS <7, or severe maxillofacial trauma.

  - **Hyperventilation:** Only to be used in acute situation to reverse intracranial HTN. Goal P_{CO_2}: 30–35 mm Hg.

- **Mannitol (Osmitrol):**

  - Indications: If there is evidence of increased ICP (as above) or mass effect with focal deficit or identified lesion, or a sudden deterioration in neurologic status.

  - Dose: emergent bolus: 1 g/kg IV (average dose 75–100 g); maintenance—0.25–0.5 g/kg q4h IV (average dose 50–75 g q4–6h)

- **Or** evacuation of surgical lesions (i.e., SDH/EDH)

- **ICP monitors ("bolts"):**

  - If the patient does not have a lesion requiring surgery, he or she may still be at risk for cerebral swelling and increased ICP requiring ICP monitoring.

  - Indications: GCS ≤8 and *either* an abnormal head CT (high or low-density lesions, EDH, SDH, contusions) *or* a normal head CT with ≥2 of the following risk factors:

    - Age >40

    - SBP <90 mm Hg

    - Decerebrate or decorticate posturing on motor exam

  - Contraindications: coagulopathy—PT/PTT must be absolutely normal and platelets >100,000.

Seizure Prophylaxis

Indications

Patients with the one of the following high-risk criteria:

- SDH, EDH

- Open depressed skull fracture

- Seizure within first 24 hrs of trauma

- GCS <10

- Penetrating brain trauma

- History of alcohol abuse

- Contusion on CT

Phenytoin (Dilantin)

- Load 18 mg/kg IV (approximately 1 g)

- Maintenance: 300 mg PO qhs, or 100 mg IV q8h, or 200 mg/tube bid

- Should stop after 7 days unless one of the following, in which case patient should be on phenytoin for 6 mos:

  - Penetrating brain injury

  - Late posttraumatic seizure (>7 days after seizure)

  - Prior seizure history

  - Patient undergoing craniotomy

SUBARACHNOID HEMORRHAGE

Etiologies for subarachnoid hemorrhage (SAH) include traumatic SAH, the most common and spontaneous SAH, of which 75–80% are related to aneurysm and another 5% are related to arteriovenous malformation.

Overall, approximately 50% of patients die within 1 mo of the initial hemorrhage from various causes, with rebleeding being the major cause of morbidity and mortality. More than two-thirds of patients who have a ruptured aneurysm successfully clipped will not return to their baseline level of function.

Symptoms

If conscious, patients will often complain that they have "the worst headache of my life," and the headache is described as though someone "struck me in the back of the head." Headache is of sudden onset and usually is accompanied by nausea, vomiting, and neck pain. Loss of consciousness is a common finding after SAH; focal cranial nerve deficits can also occur.

Coma after SAH or decline in neurologic status necessitates an evaluation for increased ICP.

The patient needs a head CT to ensure there is no surgical mass lesion (i.e., intraparenchymal hemorrhage, rebleeding of SAH, HCP), most notably HCP, which is common among SAH patients.

Evaluation

- Complete neurologic exam, including ocular exam, to look for evidence of subhyaloid or vitreous hemorrhage (known as *Terson's syndrome*).

- **Head CT scan:** Location may be as follows:

  - Anterior interhemispheric: anterior communicating aneurysm

  - Sylvian fissure: middle cerebral or posterior communicating aneurysm

  - Third and fourth ventricle: posterior fossa aneurysm, such as posterior inferior cerebellar artery aneurysm

- Lumbar puncture:

  - CT scan may be only 95% sensitive at 48 hrs; thus, lumbar puncture may be performed with high clinical suspicion to look for evidence of **xanthochromia** or frank blood. Xanthochromia is also a predictor of risk for vasospasm based on amount of blood in the cisterns.

- Cerebral angiogram is the **gold standard** for evaluation of the cerebral vasculature and should be done for all nontraumatic SAH.

- Classification and grade: Use the Hunt and Hess Classification for SAH (Table 76-1).

TABLE 76-1.
HUNT AND HESS CLASSIFICATION FOR SUBARACHNOID HEMORRHAGE

Grade	Description
0	Unruptured aneurysm
1	Asymptomatic or mild headache and slight nuchal rigidity
2	Cranial nerve palsies (III and IV), moderate to severe headache, and nuchal rigidity
3	Mild focal deficit, lethargy, or confusion
4	Stupor, moderate to severe hemiparesis, early decerebrate posturing
5	Deep coma, decerebrate rigidity, moribund

Management

Initial concerns are rebleeding, hyponatremia (CSW; see Hyponatremia), vasospasm, hydrocephalus, cardiac arrhythmia and ischemia, seizure, and deep venous thrombosis/pulmonary embolism.

Rebleeding

Rebleeding is the most preventable complication and requires that the vascular abnormality be identified and treated as quickly as possible.

- 15–20% of aneurysms will rebleed in the first 2 wks, and approximately 50% of patients will have another hemorrhage in the first 6 mos.
- Ventriculostomy and higher Hunt-Hess Scale patients have higher rates of rebleeding.

Hydrocephalus

Acute hydrocephalus is a surgical emergency.

- Occurs in approximately 10–15% of SAH patients and initially is treated with **ventriculostomy** followed by permanent shunt if hydrocephalus does not resolve.
- A small, increased risk of rebleeding exists with the placement of ventriculostomy thought to be secondary to an increase in the transmural pressure across the aneurysm wall (transmural pressure = mean arterial pressure – ICP).
- Up to 50% of patients may need permanent CSF diversion.
- Intraventricular hemorrhage increases the risk for acute hydrocephalus.

Vasospasm

- Occurs in 20–40% of SAH and can lead to ischemic stroke.
- Symptoms are gradual in onset and can include worsening level of consciousness, increased headache, and focal neurologic signs.
- Highest incidence during postbleed days 6–8 but can occur through day 17.
- Sometimes can be mitigated by keeping patients with a positive fluid status.
- Treatment includes the *HHH therapy* with *h*ypertension, *h*ypervolemia, and *h*emodilution. Usually, to start therapy, mean arterial pressures will be increased by 10–15% when vasospasm is suspected.
- Angiogram will allow for both confirmation and directed therapies, including intraarterial papaverine and balloon angioplasty.

Seizures

Seizures occur in up to 10% of patients after SAH, and prophylaxis with antiepileptic medication is standard practice. Medications:

- Decadron: 4 mg IV/PO q6h

- Phenytoin (as noted above) for seizure prophylaxis

- Nimodipine: 60 mg PO q4h

  - A calcium channel blocker, which has been shown to improve outcome in lower-grade patients

SPINAL CORD INJURIES

- 20% of patients with a major spine injury will have a second spinal injury at another level that may or may not be contiguous.

- *Spinal column instability* is defined as the inability of the spinal column under physiologic loads to prevent spinal cord and spinal nerve root injury and to prevent incapacitating deformity or pain due to structural changes.

Types of Lesions

Incomplete

Any residual function >3 segments below the level of injury

- Sensation and/or voluntary movement in the lower extremities.

- Sacral sparing, although presence of reflex alone does not qualify a patient as incomplete.

- Defined types include anterior, posterior, and central cord syndrome, and Brown-Séquard syndrome.

Complete

No residual motor and/or sensory function >3 segments below the level of injury.

Spinal Shock

- Hypotension with systolic BP usually <80.

- Transient loss of all neurologic function—flaccid paralysis and areflexia—lasting an undetermined time from weeks to months, and sometimes permanent.

- Resulting spasticity with recovery.

- Some will have no spinal reflexes on initial evaluation. If patients do not have bulbocavernosus or anal wink, then they may have spinal shock rather than a complete injury.

Evaluation

- Initial ABCs and management of possible hypotension. BP in spinal cord injury should be maintained with pressors; fluid resuscitation will be ineffective.

- Exam should include mental status, motor, sensory, and reflexes, and evaluation for *rectal tone* and *bulbocavernosus reflex/anal wink*.

- *Plain films*: cervical spine (includes posteroanterior, lateral, swimmer's view to see C7-T1 junction, open mouth odontoid) and thoracic and lumbar spine films (posteroanterior and lateral views).

- Flexion/extension films can be taken to rule out occult instability with ligamentous damage. Do not attempt with obvious fracture or in patients with neurologic deficit or subluxation >3.5 mm.

- CT/MRI: to evaluate the bony and soft tissue anatomy of the spine.

Management

- High cervical injury with diaphraghmatic paralysis may necessitate intubation, which must be done with extreme caution.

- All patients with incomplete and complete spinal cord injury are given **methylprednisolone (Solumedrol)** for 24 hrs if within 3 hrs of the injury and 48 hrs if within 8 hrs of the injury. Protocol requires 30 mg/kg IV bolus followed by an infusion of 5.4 mg/kg/hr IV.

- Traction may be required if patient is misaligned to decompress the spinal cord for cervical injuries.

- Emergent surgical decompression is generally used only in cases of incomplete lesions, with the one notable exception being central cord syndrome.

- Some surgeons will operate on complete lesions <8 hrs old in young patients, because they may have some functional recovery.

Specific Spinal Cord Injuries

Central Cord Syndrome

Central cord syndrome (CCS) is the most common injury; it usually follows hyperextension injury in the presence of cervical stenosis due to bony hypertrophy.

- Often a blow to the face or forehead.

- Can occur without fracture or dislocation.

CCS is thought to occur because the medial portion of the spinal cord is a watershed area, making it susceptible to injury from edema. The syndrome is as follows:

- Motor: Upper greater than lower, distal greater than proximal.

- Sensory: Hyperpathic pain is common, but sensory findings are varied.

- Myelopathy: Sphincter dysfunction.

CCS may be caused by disk herniation, traumatic fracture/dislocation, or congenital/degenerative narrowing of the spinal canal. Treatment includes

- Surgery, the timing of which is controversial and case-to-case dependent (unless patient with instability or continued spinal cord compression).

- Conservative therapy with soft cervical collar and physical therapy.

Anterior Cord Syndrome

Anterior cord syndrome refers to cord infarction in the territory supplied by the anterior spinal artery.

- Presentation is with paraplegia or quadriplegia if higher than C7.

- Dissociated sensory loss with loss of pain and temperature (spinothalamic) but preservation of posterior columns and thus light touch, position, and two-point discrimination.

- Must decide if case is surgical. MRI, CT, and myelogram to evaluate whether a bony fragment or disk herniation is present.

Brown-Séquard Syndrome

Spinal cord hemisection usually follows penetrating traumatic injury but may occur with tumor, disk herniation, and rarely degenerative spinal disease. It classically presents with loss of proprioception, vibration, and motor strength on the side of the lesion (posterior column, corticospinal pathways), and loss of contralateral temperature and pinprick (spinothalamic) that occurs 1–2 segments below the lesion.

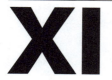

XI

Surgical Subspecialties: Orthopedic Surgery

77 Orthopedic Surgery Essentials

Raja Dhalla

KEYS FOR SURVIVAL

- Know your extremity anatomy.

- Become familiar with reading bone x-rays and describing fractures.

- Don't be afraid of "getting your hands wet." Try to practice techniques of cast and splint application, joint aspiration, traction pin insertion, common closed reductions, and measuring compartment pressures.

- Don't be afraid to ask questions.

- Develop a system for organizing patients' labs, x-rays, and coumadin logs.

- Remember to include deep venous thrombosis prophylaxis on admission and postoperative orders.

- Learn how to perform and document neurologic and vascular exams.

- Remember to read consultants' notes and follow up on their recommendations.

- Communicate with physical therapists and social workers to plan discharges.

- Try to have fun. Usually, orthopedics services are a lot less stressful than other general surgical services. Even rotations with long hours can be fun if you enjoy the work and develop a good rapport with the senior team members.

INTRODUCTION TO THE DAILY ROUTINE

Unlike general surgical and medical services, orthopedic progress notes and rounds are not routinely systems based (although spine fusion patients may be an exception to this rule). The daily exam should focus on the injured and/or postoperative extremity. A distal neurologic and vascular exam should be documented. When surgical and traumatic wounds are present, the wound appearance or dressing should be documented periodically. Unlike general surgery, orthopedic wounds are sometimes difficult to access due to overlying casts or splints. Consult a senior member of the orthopedic team as to when casts and splints should be taken down for wound checks and dressing changes.

Important pre-rounding information that an intern can help gather includes vital signs (particularly temperature), laboratory values, drain output recordings, and any recent radiographs that may be of interest to the orthopedic team. The intern should also work with the orthopedic team in organizing the x-rays of the patients on the service. Most services will require "templating" or preoperative planning before taking a patient to the OR. This often requires planning of the particular orthopedic implants to be used, as well as the surgical approach. Interns should learn some basic templating skills from senior residents and common surgical anatomy and approaches.

Almost all patients will require deep venous thrombosis prophylaxis. Regimens vary by attending surgeons and institutions. Anti-embolism stockings and sequential compressive devices are almost always ordered on orthopedic patients. If coumadin is used, the intern should keep a log of the coumadin dosing as well as the daily INR value. Most patients with orthopedic implants will require prophylactic antibiotics. Although surgeon and institution specific, this is usually a first-generation cephalosporin.

Orthopedic interns should communicate with physical and/or occupational therapists and social workers to plan discharges. Also, interns should be aware of medical and general surgical consultants' recommendations for inpatient management issues and for follow-up after hospital discharge.

78

Orthopedic Surgery: Emergencies

Raja Dhalla

When called, the following situations require immediate attention.

OPEN FRACTURES AND FRACTURES WITH ASSOCIATED NEUROVASCULAR COMPROMISE

Key Points to Remember

- Plain radiographs of the bone involved must be obtained. Usually, anteroposterior (AP) and lateral views are sufficient. However, in certain instances, additional views are necessary. Common fractures in which additional views are necessary for diagnosis and/or preoperative planning:

    - Shoulder/proximal humerus: AP, true AP, axillary view, scapular lateral (or Y) view

    - Femoral neck/intertrochanteric fractures: AP hip, cross-table lateral, AP ortho pelvis

    - Acetabular fractures: AP ortho pelvis, Judet views

    - Ankle: AP, lateral, mortise

    - Foot: AP, lateral, medial oblique. Obtain a Harris heel (axial) view if a calcaneal fracture is suspected.

- When *describing fractures*, attempt to delineate the following:

    - Fracture pattern (transverse, oblique, spiral)

    - Displacement

    - Angulation

    - Shortening

    - Comminution

- Pertinent *history* includes mechanism of injury and preinjury level of activity.

- Pertinent *exam* includes complete distal neurologic and vascular exam.

Diagnosis

Usually, plain radiographs are sufficient. However, if you suspect an occult fracture, obtain an MRI or bone scan to confirm. For hip fractures, bone scans may not be positive until 2–3 days postinjury. MRIs are positive within 24 hrs.

Initial Treatment

- Open fractures require emergent operative débridement and fixation. All patients should be NPO, given IV antibiotics according to grade, and given tetanus toxoid (if immunization is not up to date).

- Open fractures are graded I–III, with III being most severe.

  - Grade I fractures have wounds <1 cm long; give cefazolin.

  - Grade II fractures have wounds >1 cm; give cefazolin and gentamicin.

  - Grade III fractures are subdivided as follows; give cefazolin, gentamicin, and penicillin (if associated with gross tissue contamination).

    - IIIa: wound >10 cm without periosteal stripping

    - IIIb: periosteal stripping

    - IIIc: associated vascular injury

  - Closed fractures are treated based on particular bone involvement and amount of displacement.

  - When lower extremity fractures are diagnosed, consider initiating deep venous thrombosis prophylaxis with antiembolism stockings and sequential compressive devices and/or SC low-molecular-weight heparin.

Traction

Skeletal

- Involves traction of a bone via placement of a traction pin.

- Commonly used for acetabular fractures and femur fractures in which open reduction and internal fixation is delayed.

- Femoral traction pins are preferred for these conditions.

- Tibial traction pins are used for distal femur fractures.

Traction Pin Placement

- Femoral traction pin: Should be drilled from medial to lateral at the level of the superior pole of the patella, just above the medial epicondyle (to avoid injury to the popliteal vessels).

- Tibial traction pin: Should be drilled from lateral to medial just posterior and inferior to the tibial tubercle (to avoid injury to the peroneal nerve).

SEPTIC JOINTS
Key Points to Remember

- A septic joint should be suspected with history and exam demonstrating effusion, warmth, painful range of motion, tenderness, and fevers.

- Workup should include plain radiographs, CBC, ESR, CRP, and blood cultures (if febrile).

Diagnosis

- Diagnosis is confirmed with joint aspiration, which may be done by the primary physician or an orthopedics consultant. Send synovial fluid for stat Gram stain, cell count, crystals, and culture. *Do not administer antibiotics until a joint aspirate is obtained.* The patient should be NPO until the cell count and Gram stain are found to be negative for sepsis.

- Septic arthritis is generally diagnosed with a synovial fluid leukocyte count >80,000/mm^3, a positive Gram stain, or a positive culture.

- An inflammatory/autoimmune arthropathy typically has a synovial fluid leukocyte count of 10,000–50,000/mm^3 with positive crystals (for gout or calcium pyrophosphate deposition disease) and negative Gram stain and cultures.

Treatment

Operative drainage and appropriate IV antibiotics as determined by cultures. [*Neisseria* species (*gonorrhoeae* and *meningitidis*) are exceptions to the operative drainage rule, as they are highly responsive to antibiotic therapy, and operative débridement is not necessary.] Therefore, once the diagnosis is confirmed, the patient should be NPO in preparation for operative drainage. The course of antibiotics is typically 6 wks total, with the first 1–2 wks given as IV antibiotics.

Staphylococcus aureus is the most common orthopedic pathogen. In sexually active adolescents and adults, *Neisseria gonorrhoeae* has a particularly high prevalence, whereas *Salmonella* has a particularly high prevalence in sickle cell patients.

COMPARTMENT SYNDROME
Key Points to Remember

- Compartment syndromes are caused by elevated hydrostatic pressure within a fascial compartment (commonly from bleeding or swelling), leading to tissue ischemia as compartment pressure exceeds capillary pressure.

- All external circumferential dressings should be removed before examining a patient for compartment syndrome.

History

Typical history may include

- Trauma (fracture or muscle contusion)
- Ischemia
- Venous obstruction
- Massive inflammation from snake/insect bites
- Bleeding into the compartment (consider in anticoagulated patients)
- Infiltration of fluid material into a compartment (paint gun injuries)
- Tight circumferential dressings

Diagnosis

- The most specific signs and symptoms are pain out of proportion to injury, pain with passive stretch of the muscles in the involved compartment, and hard tense compartments.
- Paresthesias, pallor, pulselessness, and paralysis may or may not be present.
- The diagnosis is a clinical one. However, when clinical signs are equivocal, compartment pressures may be measured.
- Compartment pressures >30 mm Hg (or a diastolic BP–compartment pressure difference >30 mm Hg for hypotensive patients) are diagnostic for compartment syndrome.

Treatment

- The patient should be made NPO.
- Emergent fasciotomy.
- Remember that myoglobinuria can occur with compartment syndrome from muscle necrosis.

ACUTE CAUDA EQUINA SYNDROME
Key Points to Remember

- Cauda equina syndrome is an injury to the spinal canal located between the conus and the lumbosacral nerve roots that results in bowel and bladder dysfunction, saddle anesthesia, severe lower extremity neurologic deficit, and anal sphincter laxity.

- Because the cauda equina functions as the peripheral nervous system, in a complete cauda equina injury, all peripheral nerves to the bowel, bladder, perianal area, and lower extremities are lost. No bulbocavernosus, anal wink, or lower extremity reflexes will be present.

Diagnosis

- Suspect cauda equina syndrome in a patient with low back pain and the above signs and symptoms.

- Perform a complete lower extremity neurologic exam, including lower extremity strength, sensation, and reflexes. A rectal exam should also be performed to assess rectal tone and perianal sensation. Once the diagnosis is suspected, the patient should be NPO.

- Include stat AP and lateral views of the lumbar spine, as well as a stat MRI of the lumbar spine.

- If the patient has had a prior diskectomy, the MRI should be obtained with gadolinium contrast.

- If the patient has had previous spine instrumentation, obtain a CT myelogram.

Treatment

Emergent operative decompression.

79

Approach to Orthopedic Injuries

Raja Dhalla

UPPER EXTREMITY INJURIES
Shoulder/Clavicle

The clavicle is the most commonly fractured bone in the human body. 85% of clavicle fractures are in the middle third.

Treatment

Usually nonoperative, which includes a sling or figure-of-8 brace initially. Indications for open reduction and internal fixation (ORIF):

- Open injury
- Neurovascular involvement
- Floating shoulder
- Combined clavicle and glenoid neck fracture
- Skin is in danger

Acromioclavicular Joint Separation (Separated Shoulder)

Disruption of the soft tissues around the acromioclavicular (AC) joint renders the shoulder girdle unstable. The mechanism of injury is an inferior force placed directly onto the acromion, such as a fall onto the shoulder or a collision.

Classification of Acromioclavicular Separation

- Grade 1: Partial tear of the AC capsule without displacement
- Grade 2: Complete tear of the AC capsule with intact coracoclavicular (CC) ligament; <50% clavicle width displacement
- Grade 3: Complete tear of the AC capsule and CC ligament, with superior displacement of the clavicle
- Grade 4: Complete tear of the AC capsule and CC ligament, with posterior displacement of the clavicle
- Grade 5: Complete dislocation of the AC joint with detachment of the deltoid and trapezoid from the clavicle
- Grade 6: Inferior/subcoracoid dislocation of the clavicle

Treatment

Differs depending on grade of injury:

- Grades 1 and 2 are treated with a sling and early range of motion exercises.

- Grade 3 injuries are usually treated with a sling and early range of motion exercises, but surgical treatment may be selected in overhead athletes and heavy laborers.

- Surgical treatment is the standard of care for grade 4–6 injuries.

Shoulder Dislocation

- The shoulder has been displaced from its normal anatomic location inside the glenoid fossa.

- Radiographs are required, including AP, lateral, and axillary views.

- Most commonly dislocated anteriorly, the mechanism of injury is forced abduction and external rotation, which causes the humeral head to be levered out of the glenoid.

- Distal neurovascular exam is critical in shoulder dislocations, owing to the high incidence of axillary nerve injuries.

- Examine the axillary nerve for involvement of both motor and sensory components.

  - Motor exam should include asking the patient to abduct the arm. Usually, patients are unable to abduct the arm secondary to pain, but muscular contractions of the deltoid may be palpated.

  - The sensory distribution of the axillary nerve should be tested over the lateral shoulder and upper arm.

Treatment

Closed reduction in the ER:

- Conscious sedation of choice.

- Traction/countertraction: An assistant holds countertraction by placing a sheet under the axilla and around the torso of the patient. The physician then reduces the shoulder by placing traction on the arm, abduction, and gentle internal and external rotation.

- Obtain postreduction x-rays, and perform postreduction neurovascular exam.

Proximal Humerus Fracture

Mechanism of injury: usually due to a direct blow to the extremity; however, in older, osteoporotic patients, the injury can occur after falls onto the outstretched arm.

Distal neurovascular exam must be performed, because vascular injury, especially in the elderly, may occur. Neurologic deficits are not uncommon with this injury (axillary nerve); however, they are largely reversible.

Neer classification:

- Based on the degree of displacement of the four component parts: head, shaft, greater tuberosity, and lesser tuberosity.

- Displacement between two components is defined as >1 cm of translation or 45 degrees of angulation.

- Fracture is considered a 1-part fracture if there is <1 cm of translation or 45 degrees of rotation.

Treatment

Based on the Neer classification above:

- 1-part: sling and early range of motion exercises
- 2-part:

  - surgical neck: hanging arm cast or closed reduction with percutaneous pinning

  - greater tuberosity: surgically repaired if >5 mm displacement

  - lesser tuberosity: surgically repaired if >5 mm displacement

- 3-part: ORIF
- 4-part: ORIF in young patients, hemiarthroplasty in older adults (owing to increased incidence of avascular necrosis of the humeral head in 4-part injuries)

Humeral Shaft Fracture

- Usually treated nonoperatively, by functional bracing.
- Reduction is considered acceptable with <20 degrees of AP angulation, <20–30 degrees of varus/valgus angulation, or <3 cm shortening.
- Surgery is indicated in cases of open fractures, vascular injury, floating elbow, polytrauma, or pathologic fracture.
- There is a 5–10% incidence of radial nerve palsies with humeral shaft fractures. Most of these resolve without surgery. It is important, however, to perform a neurovascular exam before and after reduction to note any changes. If radial nerve function is intact and then lost after a reduction attempt, surgical exploration of the nerve is warranted.

Distal Humerus Fracture

- Includes supracondylar and epicondylar fractures.
- It is important to perform a neurovascular exam, because approximately 1 in 5 may have neural or vascular injury.

Treatment

Casting in nondisplaced fractures, with ORIF being the gold standard for treatment of displaced fractures.

Elbow Dislocation

Usually caused by a fall onto the outstretched arm, and the forearm is generally dislocated posterolaterally.

Treatment

- Closed reduction with longitudinal traction, then splint the elbow in 90 degrees of flexion.
- Ensure that the elbow is concentrically reduced by noting that the trochlea of the distal humerus is centered in the greater sigmoid notch of the ulna.

Olecranon Fracture

Usually caused by a direct blow to the proximal ulna.

Treatment

- If the fracture fragment is displaced <2 mm: Long arm splint, sling, and early range of motion exercises.
- If the fracture is displaced >2 mm: Place the patient in a long arm splint and refer for potential ORIF.

Radial Head Fracture

Caused by axial loading with the forearm in full pronation.

Treatment

- If the fracture fragment is displaced <2 mm: Long arm splint, sling, and early range of motion exercises.
- If the fracture is displaced >2 mm and/or there is a block to pronation/supination: Splint and refer for ORIF.

Distal Radius Fracture

- Classified based on the displacement and angulation of distal pieces.
- Named fracture patterns that merit discussion:
  - *Colles' fracture*: dorsal displacement and angulation
  - *Smith's fracture* (reverse Colles'): volar angulation with volar displacement
  - *Barton's fracture*: displaced intraarticular fracture with dislocation; can be volarly or dorsally displaced

- *Chauffer's fracture*: a fracture of the radial styloid

Treatment

- Treat nondisplaced fractures with a sugar-tong splint.

- For displaced fractures, a closed reduction followed by splinting is preferred.

- If an anatomic reduction cannot be achieved, the patient may require ORIF or closed reduction with percutaneous pinning in the OR.

- Because Colles' fracture is one of the most common orthopedic injuries of the upper extremity, the method for reduction of the Colles' fracture bears mentioning. Along with conscious sedation or hematoma block:

  - Disimpact the fracture with longitudinal traction and wrist extension.

  - Perform reduction via pushing the distal radius fragment volarly.

  - Stabilize the reduction with pressure on the distal fragment in pronation, flexion, and ulnar deviation, and maintain the reduction with sugar-tong casting.

Scaphoid Fracture

- Occurs after a fall onto the outstretched hand.

- Classically presents as pain in the anatomic snuffbox.

- Negative x-rays do not rule out scaphoid fracture, and patients with this clinical picture may be treated as though they have a nondisplaced scaphoid fracture.

Treatment

- Nondisplaced: thumb spica cast until union

- Displaced: owing to the high incidence of nonunion and avascular necrosis as a result of retrograde blood flow to the scaphoid (and disruption after fracture), ORIF is the treatment of choice for displaced scaphoid fractures.

Metacarpal Fracture

- Thumb metacarpal: Several named fracture patterns are described in thumb metacarpal fractures.

  - *Bennett's fracture*: Intraarticular fracture of proximal articular surface. Avulsion of a fragment of the metacarpal owing to the volar oblique ligament.

  - *Rolando's fracture*: Intraarticular, comminuted fracture of proximal articular surface.

- Treatment:
  - If nondisplaced, use a thumb spica.
  - If displaced, Bennett's fracture can be treated with closed reduction and percutaneous pinning. Displaced Rolando's fracture is treated with ORIF if not grossly comminuted, but an external fixator may be applied to grossly comminuted Rolando's fractures.
- Second through fifth metacarpal fractures:
  - Fourth and fifth metacarpal fractures are called *Boxer's fractures*.
  - Treatment:
    - Follow the rule of 40-30-20-10. For the fifth metacarpal, 40 degrees of angulation is acceptable; 30 for the fourth metacarpal, 20 for the third metacarpal, and 10 for the second metacarpal.
    - Normal rotation can be approximated by placing the fingers in passive flexion; in this position, they should all point at the scaphoid.
    - If rotation or angulation is excessive, attempt closed reduction, and if unsuccessful, perform closed reduction with percutaneous pinning.

Interphalangeal Dislocations

- Treated with closed reduction; usually stable after reduction.
- May be treated with Alumafoam splint or buddy-taping after reduction.

Distal Phalangeal Fractures

Usually treated with Alumafoam splinting.

Proximal and Middle Phalangeal Fractures

- Treated with reduction and splinting (plaster or Alumafoam) for displaced fractures.
- Splinting alone or buddy-taping alone may be used for **nondisplaced fractures.**

Gamekeeper's Thumb

- Caused by a valgus (radial) stress placed on the proximal phalanx of the thumb. This stress causes the rupture of the ulnar collateral ligament of the thumb metaphalangeal (MP) joint.
- Test the joint's stability in full extension and 30 degrees of flexion. Stress x-rays may be obtained to confirm the diagnosis.

Treatment

- Incomplete injury is treated with 4–6 wks in a thumb spica or orthosis.

- Complete injury is cause for open repair.

- In many cases, the torn ligament is displaced behind the insertion of the adductor pollicis (Stener's lesion) and will not heal without open treatment. Stener's lesion is usually present if instability is detected in full extension and 30 degrees of MP flexion.

PELVIC FRACTURES
Pelvic Ring Fractures

Suspect pelvic ring fracture in patients with

- High-energy fractures
- Abnormal lower-extremity positions
- Scrotal or labial swelling
- Free motion of the hemipelvis
- Soft tissue injury around the pelvis
- Urologic and lower extremity injuries

Management

- The goal is to determine whether the pelvis is mechanically stable. If the patient is hypotensive and not responding well to blood and fluids, consider immediate fixation of the pelvis, angiography, and embolization.

- Radiographic evaluation should include anteroposterior pelvis, inlet, and outlet views. Pelvic CT scan with 3-mm cuts can be used for fine definition of pelvic fractures.

  - Stable pelvic fractures:

    - Diastasis of the pubic rami <2.5 cm
    - Pubic rami fracture
    - Avulsion injuries
    - Transverse fracture of the sacrum and coccyx

  - Unstable pelvic fractures:

    - Diastasis of the pubic rami >2.5 cm
    - Sacroiliac dislocation or displaced fracture dislocation of the sacroiliac joint
    - Vertical shear fracture of the ileum or sacrum

Anterior Pelvic Ring Injury Management
Pubic Symphysis Diastasis

- <2.5 cm treated nonsurgically

- >2.5 cm treated surgically with plating or external fixation alone for vertically stable injuries and plating or external fixation with posterior fixation for vertically unstable injuries.

Pubic Rami Fractures

Isolated rami fractures are treated nonsurgically; however, pubic rami fractures may occur in conjunction with unstable pelvic injuries in which posterior fixation is required.

Posterior Ring Injury Management

- Sacroiliac joint dislocations require reduction and fixation with lag screw or plates.

- Sacral fracture can occur in 3 zones:

  - Zone 1: fractures of the sacral ala lateral to the neural foramina

  - Zone 2: fractures in the region of the sacral foramina

  - Zone 3: fractures of the sacral vertebral bodies, medial to the neural foramen

  - <1 cm displaced fractures are treated nonoperatively, but surgery is indicated for fractures with >1 cm displacement and those near the neural foramina with neurologic compromise.

LOWER EXTREMITY INJURIES
Hip Injuries
Acetabulum Fractures

- Usually the result of high-energy trauma, so it is important that the patient has been stabilized by the trauma team.

- Require anteroposterior pelvis and Judet views; also CT scan with 3-mm cuts through the pelvis is used to characterize the fracture accurately.

- Check neurovascular exam, especially sciatic nerve.

- Consider deep venous thrombosis prophylaxis because of the increased incidence of pulmonary emboli associated with pelvic injuries.

- Place the patient in femoral skeletal traction initially for displaced fractures (see Traction).

Treatment

- For minimally displaced acetabular fractures and fractures concentric to the hip joint: nonoperative, with protected weight bearing and early motion.

- ORIF is reserved for displaced fractures involving the weight-bearing portion of the acetabulum.

Hip Dislocation

- Suspect in high-energy trauma, including dashboard injury.

- Most commonly posterior and can be associated with posterior acetabular wall fracture.

- Check neurovascular exam, especially sciatic nerve.

Treatment

- Closed reduction.

- Helpful to have an assistant to stabilize the pelvis.

- Flex the hip to 90 degrees, apply longitudinal traction, and gently range the hip between internal and external rotation.

- Be sure to get postreduction radiographs, and recheck neurovascular status of affected extremity.

Femoral Neck Fracture

- Usually the result of a low-energy fall in the elderly.

- Patients present with the affected extremity shortened and externally rotated.

- These fractures are intracapsular and pose a significant threat to blood flow to the femoral head.

Treatment

- Preoperative: Buck's traction and medical clearance.

- Varies for different age groups and degree of displacement.

- Young patients need ORIF with three screws in all femoral neck fractures to increase the chances of preserving the native femoral head.

- Elderly patients may have ORIF for nondisplaced fractures, or hemiarthroplasty for displaced femoral neck fractures, owing to the risk of avascular necrosis associated with displaced fractures.

Intertrochanteric Fractures

- Also usually occur after a simple fall in the elderly.
- Fractures are extracapsular.

Treatment

- ORIF with dynamic hip screw for most intertrochanteric fractures.
- 95-degree blade plate or dynamic condylar screw is used for intertrochanteric fractures with reverse obliquity.

Femoral Shaft Fractures

- Generally a high-energy injury.
- There is a 5% incidence of associated femoral neck fracture; cross table lateral of the hip needed to identify a potential femoral neck fracture.

Treatment

- Intramedullary nailing is the treatment of choice, and is ideally done <24 hrs after the injury to decrease the risk of pulmonary complications, such as acute respiratory distress syndrome, fat-emboli syndrome, pulmonary embolism, atelectasis, and pneumonia.

Knee Injuries

Patella Dislocation

- While the patella normally glides smoothly through the trochlear groove, it can dislocate and usually does so laterally.
- The patient generally presents with a flexed knee and notable effusion.
- Diagnosis is confirmed with radiographs, including sunrise views.
- Treatment: Closed reduction by extending the knee and guiding the patella medially.

Knee Dislocation

- Very high-energy injury.
- Associated with severe ligamentous injury and popliteal artery injury.
- Anteroposterior, lateral, and oblique views of the affected knee are necessary.

Treatment

- Perform reduction as soon as possible.

- Perform serial neurovascular exams.
- Consider angiogram if pedal pulses are diminished.
- Obtain vascular surgery consult if popliteal artery injury is suspected.

Tibial Plateau Fracture

Usually high-energy trauma, commonly a pedestrian who is struck by a car bumper.

Treatment

- For nondisplaced or minimally displaced fractures, nonoperative management with splinting and non–weight bearing, followed by range of motion exercises.
- Treat displaced fractures with long leg splint or knee immobilizer in the ER, followed by ORIF.

Leg Injuries

Tibial Shaft Fracture

Important to maintain a high index of suspicion of compartment syndrome with tibial shaft fractures.

Treatment

- For closed reduction, <7 degrees of varus/valgus flexion/extension is acceptable.
- ≤5 degrees rotational deformity is acceptable after reduction.
- Reduction is maintained using a long leg splint.
- If there is displacement, ORIF with a tibial nail is preferred.

Pilon Fractures

- Fractures occurring at the weight-bearing surface of the distal tibia.
- Generally high-energy axial load injuries.
- High complication rate associated with soft tissue swelling and skin breakdown.

Treatment

- Treat nondisplaced pilon fractures with splinting.
- Displaced fractures must be treated with delayed ORIF (once soft tissue swelling is reduced).

Ankle Fractures

- Radiographs must include an anteroposterior, lateral, and mortise view.

- **Weber classification:**
  - Weber A: fibular fracture below or at the level of the ankle mortise
  - Weber B: oblique fibular fracture proximal to the mortise
  - Weber C: high fibular fracture above the tibial plafond, associated with syndesmotic injury

Treatment

- Nondisplaced or minimally displaced single malleolus fracture can be treated with short leg splinting, followed by casting.
- Bimalleolar fractures or displaced fractures generally require ORIF to restore the congruency of the ankle joint.

Foot Injuries

Hindfoot Injuries

- Includes injuries to the talus, calcaneus, and navicular bones.
- Uncommon, but can cause significant disruption to the joint mechanics of the foot and ankle.

Treatment

- Minimally displaced and nondisplaced fractures are treated with casting and 4–6 wks of non–weight bearing.
- Displaced fractures, especially those with significant intraarticular involvement, may be treated with ORIF.

Midfoot Injuries

- Includes injuries to the cuboid, cuneiforms, and transmetatarsal joints.

Treatment

Minimally and nondisplaced fractures can be treated with 4–6 wks of immobilization; however, displaced fractures may be repaired with ORIF.

Lisfranc's Joint

- Spans all the tarsometatarsal joints, and injuries can vary from a slight sprain to fracture dislocations.
- Injury is diagnosed via anteroposterior/lateral/oblique views, and pronation abduction stress views may illustrate the degree of instability.

Treatment

- Cast immobilization for nondisplaced and minimally displaced injuries.
- ORIF is the treatment of choice for displaced injuries.

Forefoot Injuries

Fractures of metatarsals and phalanges are commonly due to toe stubbing or other blunt trauma.

Treatment

- Nondisplaced and minimally displaced fractures of the hallux are treated with a postoperative shoe for 3–4 wks and also may be buddy-taped as needed.

- Grossly displaced fractures and displaced intraarticular fractures require reduction and possible internal fixation.

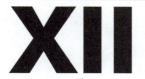

XII

Surgical Subspecialties: Urology

80 Urology Essentials

Sam B. Bhayani

Often, the intern is asked to assess urologic issues in the hospitalized patient. With rare exception, most urologic issues can be acutely managed on the hospital ward. A basic working knowledge of urologic symptoms and procedures can immensely aid the intern in successfully managing most problems. As most elderly patients are predisposed to urologic issues, the intern will quickly become familiar with these problems.

KEYS FOR SURVIVAL

- Never remove a catheter that was placed by a urologist without letting him or her know. It may be difficult to replace!

- Fever + UTI = urgency. Fever + UTI + hydronephrosis = emergency!

- Always carry a 16- to 22-Fr coude catheter to place in elderly men with benign prostatic hyperplasia.

- When dealing with hematuria, the larger the catheter, the fewer calls at night.

- *Always* check a urine culture on every urologic patient. It is the urologist's version of the ECG!

- Kidney stone = elective management. Ureteral stone = acute management.

- Testicular torsion occurs in young patients; orchitis occurs in adults.

- Bilateral hydronephrosis = urinary retention until proven otherwise.

- Be nice to the interventional radiologists; you will need them to place nephrostomy tubes for you.

- Never check a PSA test while the patient is having an acute lower urinary tract problem, as it will be falsely elevated.

INTRODUCTION TO THE DAILY ROUTINE

On the urology service, one must focus on both urologic and general medical issues during rounds. A basic assessment of the patient's vital signs, heart, lungs, and abdomen is essential. Any wound should be examined and evaluated for erythema, discharge, or infection. Most urologic patients have catheters, tubes, or drains in place. The amount and color of output from these drains should be assessed, as hematuria is common. If an indwelling catheter is draining clots, irrigation should be seriously considered. Because many urologic patients have impaired renal function, the patient's fluid status should be assessed daily. In addition to the lung exam, an assessment of peripheral edema is helpful to assess hydration status. Additionally, all medications should be checked for renal dosing if necessary.

Certain supplies are commonly used and should be readily available. The experienced intern on the urology service always carries 10-cc syringes to deflate catheter balloons, tape to secure tubes and drains, and scissors to cut drain stitches. Irrigation trays with catheter-tip syringes and saline should be present. Lubrication jelly is also commonly used.

Because many urologic patients are elderly or are discharged with indwelling catheters, the intern should communicate daily with social workers to assess home health needs. Finally, the intern must always respect the privacy of urologic patients. Because the daily exam often involves the pelvis and perineum, curtains and doors should be closed and visitors should leave before examination. Gloves should always be used.

81

Approach to Urologic Symptoms and Imaging

Sam B. Bhayani

INTRODUCTION

Urologic symptoms are subdivided into lower and upper urinary tract symptoms. Lower urinary tract symptoms are further subdivided into irritative symptoms, obstructive symptoms, and incontinence. History and symptoms are essential in determining the best imaging to use for diagnosis and evaluation.

LOWER URINARY TRACT

Lower urinary tract symptoms represent voiding complaints referable to the bladder, urethra, and prostate. The healthy adult voids 6×/day, has a bladder capacity of 300–400 mL, and is continent between voids. Although urologic disease predominates as a cause of lower urinary tract symptoms, gynecologic, GI, and neurologic etiologies should be considered if suspected. Diabetes also should be ruled out.

Irritative Symptoms

- Include frequency, dysuria, urgency, and nocturia.

- Causes of irritative voiding include UTI, hyperreflexic neurogenic voiding dysfunction, excessive fluid intake, polyuria, bladder tumor, and bladder calculi.

- Benign prostatic hyperplasia in men and cystocele in women may produce irritative symptoms or obstructive symptoms.

Obstructive Symptoms

- Include hesitancy, dribbling, weakened urinary stream, intermittency of urinary stream (stopping and starting), and straining.

- Potential causes are benign prostatic hyperplasia, urethral stricture, atonic bladder, obstructing tumor, and cystocele.

- Obstructive symptoms are usually quantified and followed with the American Urology Association symptom score (Table 81-1).

TABLE 81-1.
AMERICAN UROLOGY ASSOCIATION SYMPTOM SCORE FOR LOWER URINARY TRACT SYMPTOMS

	Not at all	Less than one time in five	Less than half the time	About half the time	More than half the time	Almost always
1. Over the last month, how often have you had a sensation of not emptying your bladder completely after you finished urinating?	0	1	2	3	4	5
2. Over the last month, how often have you had to urinate again less than 2 hours after you finished urinating?	0	1	2	3	4	5
3. Over the last month, how often have you found you stopped and started again several times while urinating?	0	1	2	3	4	5
4. Over the last month, how often have you found it difficult to postpone urination?	0	1	2	3	4	5
5. Over the last month, how often have you had a weak stream while urinating?	0	1	2	3	4	5
6. Over the last month, how often have you had to push or strain to begin urinating?	0	1	2	3	4	5
7. Over the last month, how many times did you most typically get up to urinate from the time you went to bed until the time you got up in the morning?	0	1	2	3	4	5
TOTAL						

0–7 = mild symptoms; 8–18 = moderate symptoms; 19–35 = severe symptoms.
Reprinted with permission from the American Urology Association.

Incontinence

- Unintentional leakage of urine.

- Stress incontinence is the leakage of urine from increased intra-abdominal pressure, such as coughing, exercise, or sneezing.

- Urge incontinence is the result of an uncontrolled bladder contraction associated with a strong urge to urinate.

- Overflow incontinence is secondary to a distended bladder.

UPPER URINARY TRACT

- Upper urinary tract symptoms are not specific to the urinary tract. Intraabdominal pathology should also be considered. Symptoms include flank pain, costovertebral angle pain, back pain, nausea, and abdominal pain.

- Urologic causes include nephrolithiasis, upper tract tumor, ureteral obstruction, and pyelonephritis.

- Investigation relies on imaging tailored to the history, symptoms, and patient condition.

- Imaging: CT scan, renal U/S, and IVP are the most useful imaging studies.

Noncontrast CT

- Best test to evaluate for urolithiasis.

- Also identifies hydronephrosis.

- Note that phleboliths in the pelvis are often confused for lower ureteral stones, and IVP should be considered to distinguish these entities, particularly in the absence of hematuria and hydronephrosis.

Contrast CT

- Best to evaluate renal masses, renal abscess and infection, and external compression on the urinary tract.

- Urolithiasis will not be seen, as the urinary tract will fill with contrast.

- If creatinine is >2, MRI or U/S is substituted to evaluate renal mass.

Renal Ultrasound

- Best to evaluate renal cysts.

- Can also identify hydronephrosis and grade hydronephrosis.

- CT scan is superior to U/S in the evaluation of urolithiasis and etiology of hydronephrosis.

- Advantages are relative low cost, lack of nephrotoxic contrast use, and lack of radiation.

IV Pyelography

- Preferred to evaluate hematuria, as it can identify stones and small urothelial tumors.

- May not identify renal parenchymal masses, and CT is preferred.

- Avoid in patients with a creatinine >2; retrograde pyelography is substituted by most urologists during cystoscopy.

MRI

- Useful in evaluation of renal masses.

- Also can identify renal vein invasion of renal cell carcinomas.

- Disadvantages: lack of efficacy in identifying urolithiasis and cost.

Renal Scintigraphy

- Useful to assess renal function.

- Diuretic may be administered during the exam to assess for urinary obstruction based on the washout time of the radiotracer.

82

Common Calls in Urology

Sam B. Bhayani

FOLEY CATHETER PLACEMENT
Men

Foley catheters may be difficult to place in men secondary to benign prostatic hyperplasia (BPH), urethral stricture, tortuous urethra, or prior instrumentation.

- Perform transurethral lubrication with 1% lidocaine jelly in all cases.

- Coude catheters have a curved tip so they can enter the bladder over an enlarged prostate. Typically, a 22-Fr coude is used, as it will be too large to enter a false passage. If it is too large, use a 16-Fr coude catheter.

- If catheterization with a coude is unsuccessful, bedside cystoscopy or suprapubic tube placement is indicated. Urologic consultation is indicated in these cases.

Women

Foley catheter placement in women can be difficult secondary to obesity or prior gynecologic surgery.

- Technique is based on adequate visualization of the urethra. Perform pelvic exams with legs in stirrups if possible. Evaluate any vaginal masses.

- After adequate visualization of the urethra, a 16-Fr Foley can be placed without difficulty.

- If prior gynecologic surgery precludes visualization, a suprapubic tube can be placed.

Inability to Deflate Foley Balloon

Causes include filling the balloon with saline instead of sterile water, encrustation of balloon tract, and malfunction of balloon port. Bedside treatment is usually successful.

- Balloon port is cut and removed to release balloon valve.

- A 0.038 guidewire can be passed down the balloon port to release encrustation and release balloon.

- Rarely, a smaller wire or transrectal U/S-guided puncture of the balloon is necessary.

- In women, the balloon can be pulled tightly against the urethra, and a sheathed angiocatheter may be safely passed alongside the catheter to puncture the balloon.

- Avoid overinflation and rupture of the balloon, because cystoscopy will be necessary to remove the retained balloon fragments.

HEMATURIA

Evaluate all patients with hematuria to rule out urothelial and renal tumors and urolithiasis. Consider medical renal disease, including nephritis.

Evaluation

Evaluation of hematuria includes radiographic and lab studies.

- The presence of casts or protein on urinalysis may indicate medical renal disease.

- Obtain urine culture and urine cytology in all cases.

- Radiographic exams should rule out urinary tract tumors or urolithiasis.

- IV pyelogram is the preferred test to identify urothelial lesions.

- CT scan or U/S is used to evaluate the renal parenchyma.

- If creatinine is >2, perform a retrograde pyelogram in the OR.

- Cystoscopy is essential in all patients to evaluate for lower urinary tract lesions. Usually, cystoscopy is performed in the urologist's office and is well tolerated.

Management

Acute management of gross hematuria involves hydration and correction of coagulopathy and HTN. If clots are present, place a large-bore (≥22 Fr) three-way catheter, irrigate out clots, and start continuous bladder irrigation (CBI).

- Normal saline CBI is the first-line irrigant to clear the urine.

- Aluminum CBI can also be used to chemically cauterize the bladder. As it is hypotonic, serum sodium should be followed. Aluminum toxicity can also occur in patients who have renal insufficiency.

- Aminocaproic acid (5-g IV bolus, then 1 g/hr, up to 30 g/day) is an inhibitor of plasminogen activation and acts as a procoagulant hemostatic agent. It is effective in lower urinary tract bleeding. It is contraindicated in upper urinary tract hemorrhage, as clots may cause ureteral obstruction.

- If hemorrhage cannot be controlled, consider urologic consultation for cystoscopy and bladder fulguration or formalin instillation.

- Also consider upper tract sources, such as renal tumor, ureteroarterial fistula, or unrecognized renal trauma. CT scan can aid in this diagnosis.

SCROTAL MASS
Evaluation

Scrotal masses can present acutely or chronically. Evaluation should be prompt if significant pain is present, as some cases are surgical emergencies. Evaluation strongly depends on physical exam.

- Palpate testicles for tenderness, mass, and position.

- A high-riding testicle with a transverse lie indicates torsion.

  - Hydrocele will transilluminate.

  - Varicocele may present with a "bag of worms" and occasionally testicular atrophy.

- Lab exams include UA to evaluate for infection and CBC.

- Radiographic evaluation is based on scrotal sonography, which can diagnose most etiologies but is highly operator dependent. If torsion or incarcerated hernia is strongly suspected, immediate exploration is often quicker than sonographic evaluation.

Management

- Testicular torsion is a *surgical emergency*.

  - Detorsion can be attempted bedside, but prompt exploration is essential for testicular salvage.

  - Contralateral orchiopexy should also be undertaken.

- Epididymoorchitis often presents with urinary infection and an enlarged, painful testicle.

  - Treatment is with ceftriaxone (Rocephin), 1 g IV, and azithromycin (Zithromax), 2 g PO for younger patients in whom gonorrhea is suspected.

  - In elderly patients, benign prostatic hypertrophy is the primary etiology; use *trimethoprim-sulfamethoxazole* (Bactrim) or a quinolone for 14–28 days.

- Inguinal hernia may be repaired electively. Incarcerated or strangulated inguinal hernia should receive prompt surgical evaluation.

- Testicle mass is often testicular cancer. Perform inguinal orchiectomy urgently, as these tumors have a rapid rate of growth. Draw tumor markers of alpha-fetoprotein and beta-hCG before orchiectomy.

- Hydroceles and varicoceles can be repaired electively.

RENAL MASS
Evaluation

Evaluation is based on radiographic tests.

- Asymptomatic renal masses are occasionally seen with cross-sectional imaging.

- CT scan or MRI can suggest renal cell carcinoma.

- Triple-phase CT scan is the gold standard, but MRI can be substituted if renal insufficiency is present.

- U/S is reserved for evaluation of renal cystic disease.

Differential Diagnosis

Etiologies of renal mass include

- Benign and malignant renal cysts

- Renal cell carcinoma

- Benign renal tumors

Management

- Treatment of renal masses is predominantly surgical.

- Although CT scan may be diagnostic of benign renal cysts or angiomyolipoma, in most cases of solid masses, malignancy cannot be ruled out. Renal biopsy is contraindicated, as biopsy also cannot definitively rule out malignancy and may seed tumor in the biopsy tract.

  - Undertake surgical therapy in all cases in which malignancy is suspected. The overwhelming majority of solid renal masses are malignant. Preoperative evaluation should include metastatic evaluation with chest radiograph and CT or MRI of the abdomen. Bone scan and chest and head CT may be indicated in selected cases.

  - Paraneoplastic syndromes are common with renal cell carcinoma and include hypercalcemia, liver function abnormalities, anemia, polycythemia, and hypercoagulable state. These syndromes often resolve with tumor excision.

  - Surgery can consist of radical nephrectomy with or without adrenalectomy. Partial nephrectomy is attempted with small tumors or in the setting of renal insufficiency. Laparoscopic approaches have been shown to have less postoperative morbidity than open procedures.

- Renal tumors may invade the vena cava and extend into the chest. U/S or MRI of the vena cava is preferred in selected cases to plan surgery.

KIDNEY STONES

Acute management of renal colic from kidney stones is a common problem in the ER. Most patients have been diagnosed radiographically by the time a urologic consult is called.

Presentation

- Colicky flank pain
- Abdominal pain
- Testicular pain
- Groin pain
- Microscopic or gross hematuria. Hematuria may be absent if the stone is completely obstructing the ureter.

Evaluation

- Lab exam usually reveals hematuria.
- Radiographically, most stones are diagnosed by noncontrast CT or IV pyelography. Hydronephrosis is very common in patients with ureteral stones. It does not usually denote a complete obstruction. CT can misdiagnose a pelvic phlebolith as a ureteral stone.

Management

- Treatment depends on
  - Size of stone
  - Location of stone
  - Patient's clinical appearance
- Stones in the absence of UTI or hydronephrosis are usually managed electively with lithotripsy or ureteroscopic extraction. Percutaneous nephrolithotomy is required in stones >2 cm.
- Ureteral stones can be observed for several weeks if the patient is comfortable and tolerating oral intake. Most stones <5 mm in size will pass on their own.

- If the patient cannot tolerate the ureteral stone or it is >5 mm, patients are usually treated operatively with lithotripsy, cystoscopic stent placement, or ureteroscopic stone extraction.

- Urolithiasis and urinary obstruction in the presence of febrile UTI is a surgical emergency, as patients can rapidly progress to urosepsis and circulatory collapse. Patients are usually managed with acute nephrostomy tube placement or acute decompression with a ureteral stent.

- Patients admitted with urolithiasis should be very well hydrated (2× maintenance fluids) to allow the ureters to dilate and assist in stone passage. Obtain a urine culture, and administer antibiotics if necessary.

- Patients with a solitary kidney and obstructing urolithiasis present with pain, anuria, and renal failure. Emergent decompression of the kidney with a stent or nephrostomy is essential.

HYDRONEPHROSIS

Hydronephrosis is discovered by renal imaging and is a relative indicator of urinary tract obstruction.

Presentation

Presenting signs and symptoms are variable.

- Creatinine may be elevated, particularly if the contralateral kidney has abnormal function.

- Flank pain, hematuria, abdominal pain, and fever may be present.

- Chronic urinary tract obstruction is often asymptomatic.

Evaluation

- Radiographic evaluation can determine the cause of hydronephrosis.

- Perform abdominal CT scan if extrinsic compression is suspected.

- Noncontrast CT or IV pyelogram may be performed if urolithiasis is suspected.

- Renal scintigraphy with diuretic may quantitate the degree of obstruction and can evaluate the function of the affected kidney.

Differential Diagnosis

- Hydronephrosis can be intrinsic or extrinsic to the urinary tract:

  - *Intrinsic causes* are vesicoureteral reflux, bladder outlet obstruction, urothelial tumor, or urolithiasis.

  - *Extrinsic causes* include compression from mass, trauma, or inflammatory process.

Management

- Treatment is based on relief of the obstruction.

- If the cause of obstruction is temporary (e.g., small ureteral stone), hydronephrosis can be closely followed. Place a Foley catheter in all patients with bilateral hydronephrosis to rule out bladder outlet obstruction.

- Ureteral stent can be placed cystoscopically to bypass the obstruction.

  - Stents are usually not placed in the presence of active urinary infection, as urosepsis may be induced by cystoscopic manipulation.

  - Stents may be placed in the presence of coagulopathy.

  - Stents commonly cause dysuria, pyuria, and hematuria, and should be changed q3mos.

- Nephrostomy tube may be placed if stenting is not possible. It is also the preferred method of urinary diversion if infection is present.

  - Correct coagulopathy before placement to avoid renal hemorrhage.

  - Perform nephrostogram through the nephrostomy tube to further delineate the cause of obstruction.

MALE URINARY RETENTION

Urinary retention is common in hospitalized patients or after minor surgery.

Evaluation

Diagnosis is usually apparent. Patients will have a distended suprapubic mass on exam and have lower abdominal pain. Patients may present with renal failure from long-standing obstruction.

Differential Diagnosis

Etiology is most commonly BPH; urethral stricture is also common. Treatment with anticholinergic medicines also may cause urinary retention. Bladder or prostate cancers rarely cause retention.

Management

- Treatment is based on bladder decompression:

  - A Foley catheter can be placed to drain the bladder. In the elderly male, a coude catheter may be needed (16 or 22 Fr).

  - If a catheter cannot be passed, a larger catheter should be attempted. Repeated attempts with small catheters create false passages and cause urethral injury.

  - If a catheter cannot be passed, cystoscopic placement or suprapubic tube placement is necessary.

- One-time straight catheterization probably may be attempted, but if retention does not resolve, a Foley catheter should be left in place.

- All men with retention should be started on an alpha blocker. A voiding trial should be attempted after 3–5 days.

- In the presence of renal failure, a postobstructive diuresis may occur after decompression. Patients usually make copious amounts of dilute urine until their renal medulla reestablishes concentration ability. Patients should be aggressively hydrated and electrolytes should be checked twice a day until renal function improves.

- Do not screen for PSA acutely, as it is falsely elevated in patients with retention or recent urethral instrumentation.

Benign Prostatic Hyperplasia

BPH is a condition in which the bladder outlet is obstructed by an enlarged prostate. 25–50% of men >65 are affected.

Evaluation

- Men with BPH may present with a variety of obstructive and irritative voiding symptoms. Hesitancy, weak stream, straining, urgency, frequency, nocturia, and urinary retention may be present.

- To quantify BPH, the American Urological Association has developed a symptom index (see Table 81-1).

- Physical exam may reveal a suprapubic distended bladder or an enlarged prostate.

- Perform neurologic exam to rule out voiding dysfunction secondary to neurologic illness.

- Lab studies include UA and culture, as the symptoms of BPH may coexist with infection. Prostate screening antigen may be checked to evaluate for prostate cancer, but the value can be falsely elevated with urinary retention or recent catheterization.

- Uroflowmetry or urodynamics testing may be considered by urologists to distinguish BPH from urgency or neurogenic voiding dysfunction.

Management

Therapy is tailored to the severity of the symptoms.

- *Conservative measures* are indicated in all BPH patients. Fluid restriction and elimination of diuretics and caffeinated products before travel or sleep can reduce nocturia and frequency.

- *Pharmacologic therapy* falls into two major classes of medications: alpha blockers and 5-alpha reductase inhibitors.

  - Prostatic smooth muscle responds to alpha-adrenergic stimulus. Alpha-adrenergic blockade has been shown to increase urinary flow rates and decrease symptom score by up to 30%.

    - Terazosin (Hytrin) is started at 1 mg PO qhs and titrated up to 5–10 mg PO qhs over 2–3 wks. Side effects are dose related and include orthostatic hypotension, dizziness, nasal congestion, peripheral edema, and syncope.

    - Doxazosin (Cardura) is started at 1 mg PO qhs and increased to 8 mg PO qhs over 2–3 wks. Side effects are similar to terazosin.

    - Tamsulosin (Flomax) (0.4 mg PO qhs) is a highly selective alpha blocker with fewer cardiovascular side effects, so dose titration is not necessary.

  - Finasteride (Proscar) (5 mg PO qd) is a 5-alpha reductase inhibitor that reduces intraprostatic dihydrotestosterone levels, theoretically limiting prostatic growth. Treatment is necessary for 6 mos before effects are seen. Its efficacy in treating BPH is controversial:

    - The Proscar Long-Term Efficacy and Safety Study was a double-blinded, randomized placebo-controlled trial of finasteride compared to placebo. Although a statistically significant reduction in the risk of acute urinary retention and need for BPH surgery with finasteride use over 4 years was seen, critics of the study contend that >90% of patients do not benefit from finasteride and are treated unnecessarily.

    - Recent trials show that finasteride is most effective in patients with markedly enlarged prostates and has little utility in patients with mild enlargement.

    - Finasteride, terazosin, and placebo were compared in a randomized, double-blind Veterans' Administration study trial. Finasteride was found to be similar to placebo in the treatment of BPH, whereas terazosin and the combination of terazosin and finasteride offered similar reductions in the American Urological Association symptom score as well as increases in peak urinary flow rates.

    - Side effects of finasteride include loss of libido and erectile dysfunction. Finasteride causes a reduction in prostate screening antigen. For prostate cancer screening, the patient's actual PSA is doubled and therefore is considered elevated when >2.

- Surgical therapy is the preferred treatment of severe or refractory BPH.

  - Conservative surgical therapy is available in the outpatient setting. Transurethral microwave therapy and thermotherapy have been shown to moderately improve BPH symptoms with minimal side effects.

  - Transurethral resection of the prostate is the standard surgical therapy. Patient satisfaction rates are >90%, and most patients can stop BPH medications after surgery. Side effects include retrograde ejaculation in most patients, impotence (5%), and incontinence (1%).

  - Open prostatectomy is reserved for extremely large glands in which transurethral surgery is not feasible.

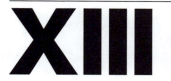

XIII Surgical Subspecialties: Plastic Surgery

83

Plastic Surgery Essentials

Benjamin W. Verdine and Aaron G. Grand

Plastic surgery is an enormous subspecialty, with most practicing surgeons dedicating themselves to but a small subset. From the intern's point of view, plastic surgery consists of wound, fracture, and laceration management. Although the remainder of the field holds some of the most fascinating, thought-provoking, and exciting aspects of all of surgery, complex reconstructive and cosmetic surgery are not extensively covered in this section.

KEYS FOR SURVIVAL

- Any amputation or questionably devascularized part is an emergency and mandates immediate notification of your senior.

- Any flap changes suggestive of venous congestion or ischemia are an emergency and mandate a call to your senior.

- Patients' wounds are rarely a source of fevers or sepsis, especially if open and draining. A more likely cause is an unidentified urinary tract infection or pneumonia.

- If you have a digital camera, use it. A photograph of a laceration or wound is better than any description.

- Make a point to learn to adequately describe x-rays (comminution, angulation, displacement, etc.).

- Try your best to make it to the OR. Plastic surgeons do things that other specialties think are crazy (and some of them probably are).

- Use your seniors to answer questions. This may be your only exposure to plastic surgery, and a lot of the experience comes from the field.

INTRODUCTION TO THE DAILY ROUTINE

In some sense, plastic surgery rounds are like most surgery rounds, because it is important to review vitals, inputs, outputs, chemistry labs, culture results, and medications. However, each of these steps takes on special importance depending on the clinical situation with respect to plastic surgery. Fevers may or may not necessitate looking at a wound, depending on the procedure and clinical situation. For instance, a fever on postoperative day 1 (or 2, or 3) would not be cause for removing a skin graft dressing. Inputs and outputs must be followed closely, because there may be many drains in place, and the outputs and timing of each dictate if and when each is removed. Many patients have procedures performed in the setting of infection, and so current culture results and antibiotic sensitivities are extremely important. Those results can dictate timing of discharge, as well as the need for home nursing services. Also, don't forget the need for ancillary services, such as physical therapy, occupational therapy, and social services for discharge planning and comprehensive care.

Paramount to plastic surgery rounds, though, are the dressing changes. The rounding cart should be stocked with all topical gels, nonadherent dressings, dry dressings, tapes, and wraps and casting supplies, etc., for the day. Rounds can be prolonged significantly if even one item is missing at each patient's bed. The easiest way to remember what is needed is to review each dressing change in your mind and have a well-stocked cart.

Common Calls
in Plastic Surgery

84 Facial Fractures

Benjamin W. Verdine and Aaron G. Grand

OVERVIEW

- Facial fractures most often occur in the setting of blunt trauma, usually an assault or a motor vehicle crash. Rarely, these fractures are associated with penetrating injury to the head or face.

- In all cases, perform a full trauma evaluation to assess associated injuries, specifically intracranial, cervical spine, chest, or abdominal trauma.

- Facial fractures are rarely life threatening, although early repair (within 1 wk) of the injury allows the greatest ease of returning previous appearance and function to the patient.

HISTORY

- Key points to elicit include any prior facial fractures or surgeries.

- Also ask about and document any change in visual acuity, new onset of diplopia, subjective change in dental occlusion, or loss of any dentition.

PHYSICAL EXAM

The physical exam consists first of observation.

- Fractures often underlie such superficial injuries as laceration, swelling, or ecchymosis.

- Take care to identify the location and depth of any lacerations, as there may be underlying open fractures or complex lacerations involving deeper musculature or intraoral or intranasal components.

The next component includes palpation of all bony structures, specifically the orbital rims, maxilla, mandible, and nasal bones.

- Document any crepitence or step offs.

- Place a gloved hand in the oral cavity and run it along the mandible and maxilla to assess for any intraoral fractures and to assess tooth root involvement.

- Rock the maxilla and midface back and forth while stabilizing the forehead to test for any instability.

Examine the nose for any rhinorrhea (indicating fracture with communication intracranially) or a nasal septal hematoma, which should be drained immediately to prevent nasal septum necrosis.

LAB EVALUATION

Labs should include standard preoperative lab tests:

- CBC
- Electrolytes
- Coagulation studies
- Type and screen

IMAGING

- The current radiographic exam of choice is a facial CT scan with 2- to 3-mm cuts in the axial, coronal, and sagittal planes; true coronal cuts are desirable but not always attainable in this patient population initially due to inability to clear the cervical spine. In these cases, perform coronal reconstruction of axial images.

- If there is any question of a mandibular fracture, obtain a Panorex. This achieves adequate imaging of the mandible and tooth roots with the exception of the condyles, which can be imaged with plain films.

MANAGEMENT

- Immediately place patients on broad-spectrum antibiotics to prevent infection. If there is any intraoral communication with a fracture, also place the patient on chlorhexadine gluconate mouthwash.

- The need for operation depends on the anatomy and degree of displacement of fractures.

Frontal Sinus Fractures

- Anterior table fractures with no or minimal displacement may be observed.

- Even anterior table fractures with significant displacement may be observed, provided there is no occlusion of the sinus and the patient understands the final cosmetic result. Repair entails exposure through a coronal incision and reduction with plates and/or wires.

- Posterior table fractures with no or minimal (<1 cortical thickness) displacement and no signs of intracranial injury may be observed, although this is controversial.

- If there is any evidence of intracranial injury (cerebrospinal fluid rhinorrhea) or any significant displacement, carry out repair in conjunction with neurosurgical colleagues, because a frontal craniotomy and dural repair may be required. If the posterior table is unable to be used for repair, obliteration and cranialization of the frontal sinus may be required.

Nasal Bone Fractures

- Nasal fractures that are nondisplaced or minimally displaced require no therapy.

- Displaced nasal fractures may produce cosmetic and functional deficits and should be reduced. Most are amenable to closed reduction and nasal packing, which controls bleeding, prevents formation of a septal hematoma, and splints and supports reduced fragments. Beware of possible development of toxic shock with packing. An alternative to nasal packing is Doyle splints.

- Indications for rhinoplasty and/or septoplasty include failed attempts at closed reduction, a patient with premorbid nasal airway obstruction, or deformity secondary to a nasal septal hematoma.

Orbital Fractures

- Orbital fractures that are minimally displaced with no signs of entrapment may require no therapy.

- Indications for surgery include any evidence of muscle entrapment, either radiographically or clinically via forced duction test (grasping of muscular insertion of a rectus muscle and demonstrating restriction of motion), or a fracture with displacement, which may result in enophthalmos.

- The goals of surgery are to restore normal bony structure to the orbit and return all soft tissue contents to within the orbit.

- The location and number of fractures dictate the surgical incisions and approach to the patient. Options and their respective exposures include

  - Subciliary: lateral, medial, floor

  - Mid-lid: lateral, medial, floor

  - Transconjunctival: lateral, medial, floor

  - Lateral brow: lateral, roof

  - Medial canthal: medial, nasal bones

  - Intraoral: inferior rim, maxilla, zygoma

  - Bicoronal: all walls

- Reconstruction is carried out with bone grafts or synthetic materials (titanium or bioabsorbable).

Zygoma Fractures

- Zygomatic fractures range from nondisplaced, to displaced arch or body, to complex "tripod" or "quadrapod" fractures. They include all attachments of the zygoma to the remainder of the skull (zygomaticofrontal, zygomaticotemporal, zygomaticomaxillary, and zygomaticosphenoidal sutures).

- Indications for operation include clinical or radiographic evidence of displacement or instability.

- Repair of an isolated arch fracture may be performed percutaneously or through a "Gillies approach," which involves a temporal incision above the hairline and elevation of the fragment by placing an instrument under the superficial layer of the temporalis muscle.

- Repair of complex fractures involves incisions as listed under Orbital Fractures above to expose the needed region and reduction with internal fixation.

Maxillary Fractures

Tend to occur along fault lines that correspond to LeFort fractures. All require fracture of the pterygoids.

- LeFort I refers to a transmaxillary fracture that goes through the maxilla at the level of the piriform rim.

- LeFort II refers to a fracture that runs across the anterior maxilla to the inferior orbital rim and through the nasal processes of the maxilla and the nasofrontal junction.

- LeFort III is complete craniofacial dissociation, with separation at the frontozygomatic suture, nasofrontal junction, medial orbital wall, orbital floor, and zygomatic arch.

- Unilateral fractures or bilateral fractures with minimal displacement may be treated with intermaxillary fixation.

- Surgery is indicated for all other fractures. The goal is restoration of aesthetics and function, specifically occlusion.

- Repair consists of intermaxillary fixation, with internal fixation of the maxilla with other craniofacial bones. Any significant displacement of orbital bones in conjunction with a maxilla fracture mandates exploration. Complex fractures may require external fixation before plating or bone grafting.

Mandibular Fractures

- Mandibular fractures are multiple in nature most of the time. Therefore, if one fracture is evident, perform a diligent search with adequate radiographs (Panorex, CT scan with reconstruction, plain films) to rule out additional fractures.

- Most mandible fractures *may* be treated with maxillomandibular fixation (MMF) for 4–8 wks. MMF is achieved by the placement of arch bars or Ivy loops; then, wire or elastic is used to provide fixation. Proper occlusion must be achieved at the time of fixation, because it is one of the major goals of fracture repair. Arch bars have the added benefit of providing fixation to any alveolar fragment fractures. Ivy loops are useful when a patient has fewer teeth, because they only require two adjacent teeth to place. In either case, adequate fixation must be achieved to prevent nonunion.

- Symphyseal and parasymphyseal fractures require compression plates to adequately reduce, in addition to MMF. This region is usually exposed through an intraoral incision at the gingivo-buccal sulcus, with care taken to preserve the mental nerve (foramen is at the second mandibular premolar).

- Condylar fractures are generally treated with 2–4 wks of MMF. The time of fixation is decreased to prevent possible temporomandibular joint changes. Inability to achieve adequate occlusion or dislocation of the condyle is an indication for open reduction.

85 Decubitus Ulcers

Benjamin W. Verdine and Aaron G. Grand

OVERVIEW

Pressure sores, or decubitus ulcers, are commonly seen in debilitated patient populations, although this is not always the case. They present a challenge to plastic surgeons and all medical staff.

Contrary to the name, pressure is but one factor in the formation of these lesions, which often go on to form chronic and costly problems. Understanding the underlying pathophysiology is important to prevent formation or progression, identify lesions early to institute therapy, and treat existing lesions.

HISTORY

Usually, an underlying condition contributes to lesion formation:

- *Altered sensation:* diabetes, peripheral neuropathy, spinal cord injury, decreased mental status

- *Altered mobility:* spinal cord injury, general medical debilitation, decreased mental status, myopathy, arthritis or joint disease, cerebrovascular event

- *Nutritional status:* poor intake, malabsorption, poor dietary habits

- *Increased potential for infection:* diabetes, fecal or urinary incontinence, prolonged antibiotic use, immunosuppression

PHYSICAL EXAM

Several general principles must be addressed. The patient's overall medical condition, general nutritional status, sensation, and mobility status are a few.

- Perform a diligent search for pressure ulcers. A person who has a lesion in one area has an increased likelihood of additional unidentified or early-stage lesions. The posterior scalp, scapular spine, thoracolumbar spine, sacrum, ischium, greater trochanter, and heel are common locations, but additional areas are possible depending on the patient's situation.

- In addition to documenting the location of any lesions, note the stage of each lesion (Table 85-1).

TABLE 85-1.
DECUBITUS ULCER STAGING

Stage	Description
I	Nonblanchable erythema of intact skin
II	Partial-thickness skin loss involving epidermis or dermis
III	Full-thickness skin loss with subcutaneous tissue involvement
IV	Full-thickness skin loss with deep structure (fascia, tendon, joint capsule, bone) involvement

LAB EVALUATION

Standard labs include a CBC, electrolytes, and nutritional assessment (e.g., albumin, prealbumin, total protein).

IMAGING

- Reserve imaging for determination of osteomyelitis.

- Initially, take plain films of the region to look for cortical destruction.

- Other studies include MRI, CT, and nuclear medicine bone scans.

MANAGEMENT

Nonoperative

- Minimization of pressure should be a primary concern. This includes scheduled turning (usually q2h, side to side) and the institution of a low-pressure bed (e.g., Kin-Aire, Clinitron).

- Take care to minimize shear and frictional forces, which are often overlooked, by training the patient and medical staff in transfers from bed to wheelchair or chair, as well as static positioning.

- Optimization of nutritional status should be undertaken with a dietitian. The patient may require supplemental drinks to maintain necessary caloric and protein requirements. If the patient is unable to comply with a regimen, enteral feeding tubes or even parenteral nutrition may be necessary. Address dietary vitamins (e.g., vitamins C and A), as well as trace cofactors (e.g., iron, zinc, magnesium, and copper).

- Infection prevention is an important adjunct to any pressure sore care. Diabetes must be strictly controlled, with the institution of insulin if diet and oral agents are unable to control glucose levels. Diversion of urinary and/or fecal stream may be necessary in some situations to prevent constant soilage and moisture to wounds. Once infection has set in, treatment with IV and topical antibiotics and frequent dressing changes may be necessary.

- Enact meticulous skin care. A member of the health care team or the patient must clean and inspect all lesions daily. Depending on the stage and depth of the lesion, moistures, barrier creams, wet-to-dry dressings, and protective dressings may be indicated.

- Nonoperative care of lesions, which optimizes the environment so that the body can heal itself or prevent a lesion from progression, can be a lengthy process, and the recurrence rate is high.

Operative

- When the decision is made to proceed to operative management, discussions with the patient and family must underscore that surgical correction is not a cure. Surgery will not change the underlying process that led to lesion formation, so unless all nonoperative principles are followed, the recurrence risk is high.

- Do not undertake surgical intervention for trivial lesions, because each operative procedure carries risks and limits future reconstructive possibilities.

- The first goal of surgical management is to remove all nonviable and infected tissue. The lesion visible on the skin is often the "tip of the iceberg" in pressure sores, with a conical region of underlying tissue involvement. The amount of tissue to remove is a clinical decision, but débridement often is carried back to bleeding tissue.

- To reduce recurrence, some surgeons resect a portion of the underlying bone to remove the underlying pressure point and redistribute pressure in the region. Take care to limit débridement and prevent skeletal instability, and not to endanger other important structures, such as vasculature or nerves.

- The final goal of surgery is to provide wound closure, using the "reconstructive ladder" (Table 85-2). This ranges from primary wound closure (not usually a viable option, because undue tension is placed on the closure, further inhibiting blood flow) to placement of a myocutaneous or fasciocutaneous flap.

- Details of flap selection are not covered in this chapter, but options for closure of various lesions include

  - Ischial: posterior thigh random flap, inferior or superior gluteal rotational flap, or thigh myocutaneous flap

  - Sacral: inferior or superior gluteal rotational, advancement, or turnover flap

  - Trochanteric: tensor fascia lata musculocutaneous flap

TABLE 85-2.
RECONSTRUCTIVE LADDER (LISTED LEAST TO MOST COMPLEX)

Procedure	Description
Secondary intention	Letting a wound granulate with dressing changes
Primary closure	Suturing the wound closed
Skin grafting	Moving skin from one site (donor) to another (recipient), with nutrition to the graft supplied by the recipient
Local flaps	Surgically mobilized tissue that maintains its original blood supply
Distant tissue transfer	Flaps that require mobilization and transfer to defect site, but still original blood supply
Free tissue transfer	Flaps that have their blood supply reanastamosed near the recipient site

86

Hand Trauma

Benjamin W. Verdine and Aaron G. Grand

OVERVIEW

- Hand trauma can devastate patients in many ways. The patient has to recover from the initial trauma but also must learn to function with any longer-term disability that results.

- The physician's ability to perform an adequate physical exam and identify potential injuries is imperative.

- Hand surgery is an extensive field that is only touched on in this chapter.

HISTORY

Important points to elicit are the mechanism and timing of injury, hand position at the time, hand dominance, and occupation.

PHYSICAL EXAM

- Initial inspection should include exam of injured and uninjured hands, looking for any deformity and swelling, and resting position of the hand.

- Assess vascularity via capillary refill, color, temperature, and presence or absence of radial and ulnar pulses.

- Perform an Allen's test as follows:

  - The patient clenches his or her fist.

  - Apply pressure to the radial and ulnar arteries

  - Open the patient's hand. Pressure is released over one of the arteries; inspect the palm with respect to return of color. Repeat the test with pressure released over the other artery. Equal time and filling of the palm indicates intact and functional palmar arches.

- Motor testing evaluates tendon and nerve integrity.

  - Test flexor digitorum profundus by stabilizing the proximal interphalangeal joint in extension and having the patient flex at the distal interphalangeal joint.

- Test flexor digitorum superficialis by blocking all other fingers in full extension before asking the patient to flex at the proximal interphalangeal joint.

- Test extensor tendons by having the patient extend each finger individually.

- Sensory testing involves careful examination of 2-point discrimination on the palmar aspect of both radial and ulnar sides of the digits and comparison to the uninjured hand. Normal 2-point discrimination is 2–6 mm at the distal tip of the digit. Light touch is used to assess the sensation on the dorsum of the patient's hand and forearm.

- The skeletal exam involves palpating for any tenderness or deformity of the bones. Joint integrity is assessed by stressing the ligaments and noting any instability, crepitus, or pain. Any suspicion of fracture or dislocation requires appropriate radiographic studies.

LAB EVALUATION

Include standard preoperative lab studies in the event that the patient requires operative repair.

IMAGING

Imaging should be directed by the injury. In general, acquire multiple views of the injured region as well as the joint above and below the injury.

MANAGEMENT
Fractures

- Most can and should be reduced in the ER using a combination of local anesthesia and conscious sedation.

- Splint, even if the patient will be going to the OR, because a well-constructed splint limits potential bleeding and further damage, and provides comfort to the patient.

- In general, a "position of function" splint may be placed for most hand injuries that includes neutral thumb position, interphalangeal joints in extension, with metacarpophalangeal and wrist flexion. This splinting places ligamentous structures in their longest position and minimizes stiffness should immobilization be required to treat the fracture.

- After reduction, take radiographs (while splinted) to confirm adequate fracture reduction.

- Operative repair is needed for failed closed reduction, open fractures, large soft tissue deficits, or intraarticular component.

TABLE 86-1.
FLEXOR TENDON ZONES

Flexor tendon zone	Anatomic location
I	Between the insertion of FDP and FDS tendons
II	Between the insertion of FDS and A1 pulley
III	Between the A1 pulley and the carpal tunnel
IV	Within the carpal tunnel
V	Proximal to the carpal tunnel

FDP, flexor digitorum profundus; FDS, flexor digitorum superficialis.

Tendon Injuries

Flexor Tendon

Any laceration to the palmar surface of the hand should raise suspicion of a flexor tendon laceration. Perform and document specific testing of the flexor digitorum profundus (FDP) and flexor digitorum superficialis (FDS) tendons, as well as the function of any distal neurovascular structures. In addition, weakened flexion against resistance should raise questions as to a partial laceration to the tendon.

- Initial management includes irrigation and closure of lacerations, and placement of a dorsal splint in the position of function (with the exception of metacarpophalangeal flexion, which should be 90 degrees to minimize stress on the flexor tendons).

- Rarely, if ever, should repair of a flexor tendon be attempted outside of the OR or by any surgeon not trained in hand surgery. Refer the patient to a hand surgeon immediately, as delay can complicate or even compromise further care and rehabilitation. Explain to the treating surgeon the location of the laceration (Table 86-1) and any functional deficits.

Extensor Tendon

Examine in a similar fashion as to flexor tendon repair; however, associated nerve damage is less frequent. Extensor damage requires referral to a hand surgeon, although some limited repairs may be performed in the ER by trained individuals. Extensor zones are listed in Table 86-2.

- *Zones I and II:* Typical injury is from forced flexion of the finger, resulting in a "mallet finger." Obtain radiographs to rule out avulsion fracture fragment. Most injuries may be treated with a distal interphalangeal extension splint for 6 wks, followed by a dynamic splint. Operative repair is indicated for open injuries or large avulsion fragments.

- *Zone III:* Results in a boutonniere deformity (proximal interphalangeal flexion, distal interphalangeal hyperextension) if not prop-

TABLE 86-2.
EXTENSOR TENDON ZONES

Extensor tendon zone	Anatomic location
I	At the DIP joint
II	Over the middle phalanx
III	At the PIP joint
IV	Over the proximal phalanx
V	At the MCP joint
VI	Over the metacarpals
VII	At the carpal joints
VIII	Over the distal radius and ulna

erly treated. Repair and splint open lacerations. Reduce and splint associated fracture dislocations.

- *Zone IV:* Injuries are usually partial lacerations because of the tendon's width at this level. An isolated lateral band or central tendon lesion can be repaired primarily with splinting and subsequent therapy. Partial lacerations need not be repaired, just splinted.

- *Zone V:* Commonly the location for a "fight bite," from the patient's fist striking another person in the mouth. If the person relays such a history, take the patient to the OR for extensive tendon and joint space exploration, as a missed injury can result in devastating bone and joint destruction. After débridement and irrigation, repair the tendon and close the wound. Place the patient on antibiotics to cover oral flora. Splinting in extension has been traditional therapy, although early passive motion splints have become more popular to limit tendonous adhesions.

- *Zones VI and VII:* Treat and splint as in zone V.

HAND EMERGENCIES
Amputation

Important information to gather about any amputation includes the level, mechanism, and timing of the amputation.

Level

Distal fingertip injuries are best managed by primary closure, using advancement flaps or skin grafts to cover the defect. More proximal amputations may be managed by shortening and rounding the bone (with care taken not to leave any exposed joint capsule), with identification and proximal transsection of nerve and tendon. Replantation is reserved for amputation of the thumb or multiple fingers, or amputation at the metacarpal, wrist, or forearm level, although there is variance among surgeons. Multiple levels of amputation are considered a contraindication.

Mechanism

Crush or degloving injuries are not amenable to replantation. A mechanism that includes contamination may require débridement of the amputated part, as well as the recipient. Perform radiographs of the amputated part and recipient. If a patient is to be transferred for replantation, wrap the amputated part in saline-moistened gauze and place it in a plastic bag; place the bag in a bath of ice and water (not saline, which depresses the mix's freezing point and can lead to frostbite of the digit).

Timing

>12 hrs' ischemia for a finger or 6 hrs' ischemia for a proximal limb is a **contraindication** to replantation.

Repair goes in the following order: bony stability, tendon repair, artery repair, vein repair, nerve repair, skin.

Compartment Syndrome

An increased tissue pressure within a fascially bounded compartment threatens the viability of nerve and muscle within the compartment and potential ischemia distal to the compartment. The syndrome is usually encountered in blunt or crush injuries, burns, or reperfusion injury, although it can be seen with penetrating injury or acute infection.

- Suspicion should be highly based on history, and serial exams should be carried out to look for paresthesias, paralysis, pain with passive motion, or increased tightness of the compartment.

- Diagnosis by measuring a compartment pressure >30 mm Hg or a differential pressure (diastolic pressure – compartment pressure) <30 mm Hg.

- Treatment includes elevation and mannitol administration, although true therapy is fasciotomy of the involved compartments. Leave these open and either close or skin graft them when the acute episode subsides.

Flexor Tenosynovitis

- Infection of the tendon sheath, usually seen after a puncture wound to the palm. Diagnosis is made by the classic Knavel's four cardinal signs of tenosynovitis:

  - Finger held in flexion

  - Fusiform or symmetric swelling of the finger

- Pain with passive extension of the finger

- Pain along the tendon sheath

- Give broad-spectrum IV antibiotics, although most cultures are negative due to prior initiation of antibiotic therapy.

- Diagnosis should prompt operative incision and drainage with extensive irrigation along the sheath. Usually, a catheter is placed in the tendon sheath for continuous irrigation.

- Late diagnosis or improperly treated tenosynovitis can lead to tendonous adhesions or rupture, bone or joint destruction, and ultimately amputation.

High-Pressure Injection Injuries

These deceivingly small injuries with paint or grease may rapidly progress to hand- or extremity-threatening emergencies with poor outcomes. The entry point receives a tremendous amount of kinetic energy. The substance injected usually has a significant degree of penetration and starts a cascade of inflammation, edema, and compression with compartment syndrome. Treatment is immediate exploration with excision of the injection site, decompression of involved fascial planes, and removal of nonviable tissue and foreign material, with irrigation, antibiotics, and delayed closure.

Procedures

More information about consent can be found in Chap. 16, Consent.

1

Nasoenteric Tube Placement

Jeremy Goodman

NASOGASTRIC TUBES

NG tubes are usually 30–40 in. long and made of plastic or silicone. They come in various diameters, with the most common adult sizes being 12, 14, 16, and 18 French. The distal end of the tube is marked every 10 cm with a black ring. Most tubes also incorporate a radiopaque stripe that can easily be identified on x-ray.

NG tubes may be single or dual lumen. Dual-lumen tubes are also known as *sump tubes*. The sump port is often blue, whereas the main tube is clear. The significance is discussed below.

Supplies

1. NG tube
2. Water-soluble lubricant
3. Catheter tip syringe
4. Adhesive tape
5. Cup of water and straw

Procedure

1. Have the conscious patient sit up with the neck flexed, if possible.
2. Allowing the patient to sip small amounts of water through a straw facilitates passage of the tube.
3. Lubricate the tip of the tube with a water-soluble lubricant.
4. Pass the tube through a nostril and into the nasopharynx. Any resistance is an indication to withdraw the tube and try again through the other nostril.
5. Encourage the patient to swallow the tube while you advance it into the stomach. Advancing the tube until only one or two black rings are left outside the nose is usually sufficient.
6. Tube position can be confirmed several ways:
   a. Place your stethoscope over the patient's stomach and rapidly inject approximately 50–60 mL of air into the tube with the syringe. Auscultation of a gurgling sound indicates proper positioning.
   b. Aspirates can be checked for pH, but remember that a patient on acid suppressive therapy may not have an acidic gastric pH.
   c. Finally, an upper-abdominal x-ray or chest x-ray may be obtained to verify placement of the tube. **Always check an x-ray before initiating feedings per NG tube.**

If suction is to be applied to evacuate the stomach, consider the type of NG tube. Single-lumen tubes should be placed to low intermittent wall suction. The intermittent nature of the suction prevents the tip from continuously sucking on gastric mucosa should it lie against the stomach wall. The dual-lumen, or sump, tube reduces this possibility by drawing air in through the sump port if the main lumen lodges up against the stomach wall. Therefore, dual-lumen NG tubes may be placed to low continuous wall suction. The blue sump port should never be capped or knotted.

NG tubes may clog if not properly maintained. If a tube becomes clogged, gently flush the main lumen with water or saline. Air can also be injected into the sump port to help unclog a dual-lumen tube. Leaving a nonfunctional tube in a patient's nose is dangerous; fix it or remove it.

NASODUODENAL TUBES

The nasoduodenal tube is placed in a similar manner to the NG tube, with the goal being postpyloric placement of the tip. If not contraindicated, giving the patient metoclopramide (Reglan), 10 mg IV approximately 30 mins before insertion, may facilitate postpyloric placement. Remove the wire once the tube has been placed. Confirm proper positioning with an abdominal x-ray before use. Note that due to the small lumen of these tubes, crushed medications should not be given through them.

2 Arterial Puncture

Jeremy Goodman

Arterial puncture is used for obtaining samples for ABG and arterial chemistry determinations. As a last resort, general blood tests and blood cultures may be drawn from an artery if no venous access is possible.

SUPPLIES

1. ABG syringe (heparinized)
2. Alcohol or iodine swab
3. Gauze
4. Bandage
5. 1% lidocaine with syringe and 27-gauge needle (optional)
6. Transport container with ice
7. Sterile gloves

PROCEDURE

1. Palpate the arterial site (Fig. A2-1A). The radial artery should be your first choice, with the femoral and brachial arteries as backups.

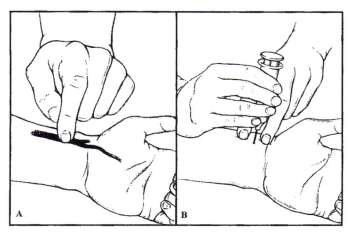

FIG. A2-1.
Arterial puncture. **A:** Palpating the artery. **B:** Stabilizing the artery with two fingers and puncturing in between.

2. Prepare the site with alcohol or iodine and allow it to dry.
3. Anesthetize the skin over the puncture site with lidocaine.
4. Palpate the artery again (Fig. A2-1B), and advance the needle at a 60- to 90-degree angle until blood is encountered. Some blood gas syringes are self-filling and do not require back pressure on the plunger. Others require gentle aspiration.
5. Obtain ≥1 mL of blood.
6. Withdraw the needle and apply the gauze with firm pressure for ≥5 mins.
7. Expel any air from the syringe, and place it on ice for transport to the blood gas laboratory.

3 Arterial Cannulation

Jeremy Goodman

Arterial catheters may be placed for real-time, invasive monitoring of BP or in anticipation of frequent ABG sampling.

SUPPLIES

1. Arterial line set or 20-gauge, 1.25- to 2-in. catheter-over-needle
2. Guidewire
3. Povidone-iodine
4. 1% lidocaine
5. 3- or 5-mL syringe with 27-gauge needle
6. 2-0 or 3-0 silk suture and needle holder
7. Gauze/sterile dressing
8. Sterile gloves and drapes
9. Armboard
10. Gauze roll
11. Tape
12. Arterial line setup, usually done by nurse (pressure tubing, transducer, heparinized saline on pressure bag)

PROCEDURE

1. The radial artery is the most frequently used site, although the femoral, axillary, and dorsalis pedis arteries may also be cannulated.
2. Before cannulating the radial artery, most authors recommend performing an Allen's test.
   a. Compress the radial and ulnar arteries.
   b. Have the patient pump his or her fist several times to exsanguinate the skin.
   c. Release the ulnar artery and watch for blood return to the hand.
   d. Blood return within 6 secs signifies a negative test and therefore an intact palmar arch. If the Allen's test is positive, most recommend not cannulating that radial artery.
3. Fasten the forearm to the armboard with a gauze roll placed under the wrist.
4. Prepare the skin overlying the artery with povidone-iodine and allow it to dry.
5. Anesthetize the skin over the puncture site with lidocaine. Always draw back before injecting to make sure you are not inside a blood vessel.

6. Palpate the artery, and insert the needle at a 30- to 45-degree angle with the bevel up until a flash of blood is encountered.
7. Once the blood flash is encountered, lower the needle slightly and advance another 1–2 mm.
8. If using an arterial line set or separate guidewire, advance the wire through the needle and into the artery. Then advance the catheter over the wire.
9. If using a catheter-over-needle assembly, advance the catheter over the needle.
10. While compressing the radial artery proximally to prevent bleeding, withdraw the needle and/or wire, and attach the pressure tubing to the catheter hub.
11. Suture the catheter to the skin with 2-0 or 3-0 silk sutures.
12. Apply a sterile dressing.

4

Central Venous Access

Emily R. Winslow

Indications for the placement of a central venous line include the following:
1. Inadequate peripheral IV access.
2. Need for measurement of central venous pressures.
3. Need for administration of medications that can only be given centrally.
4. Need for administration of TPN.
5. Need for long-term outpatient venous access.

After determining that a central venous line is, in fact, needed, the next major decision is where to place it. Central lines are commonly placed in three major locations. These include the internal jugular (IJ), subclavian, and femoral veins. The risk of line infection for subclavian lines is one-half that of IJ or femoral lines. Therefore, our preference in elective situations is to place a subclavian line in all patients who do not have a contraindication.

SUBCLAVIAN LINE CONTRAINDICATIONS

- Coagulopathy: Due to risk of uncontrolled bleeding into chest.

- Poor pulmonary reserve: Due to risk of intolerance of pneumothorax.

- End-stage renal disease: Due to risk of subclavian stenosis interfering with future dialysis access placement.

- Altered anatomy: Previous surgery (carotid-subclavian bypass).

- Known subclavian thrombosis or stenosis: Inability to pass catheter.

FEMORAL LINE CONTRAINDICATIONS

- Known pelvic or inferior vena cava thrombosis.

- Altered anatomy: Prior arterial bypass (vein harvesting).

- Groin skin infection.

- Ambulating patient: Relative contraindication.

INTERNAL JUGULAR CONTRAINDICATIONS

- Known contralateral carotid occlusion: Cannot risk compressing the only patent carotid artery.

- Recent ipsilateral carotid surgery.

- Known thrombosis or stenosis of IJ.
- Tracheostomy: Relative contraindication.

PLACEMENT OF SWAN-GANZ CATHETER

When a Swan needs to be placed through the central venous access device (a Cordis or introducer), carefully consider the position of the central venous line. It is easiest to pass the Swan through a right IJ approach, given the relatively straight path to the right atrium. However, the left subclavian is also possible and is thought of as the second most desirable location. If the Swan must be placed emergently, we suggest starting with the right IJ. However, if more time and adequate experience are available, the left subclavian route is also an acceptable initial site.

SUPPLIES

1. Central venous line kit (either a Cordis or multi-lumen kit). This should include
   a. Small-gauge needle and syringe
   b. Larger-bore needle and syringe
   c. Guidewire
   d. Catheter
   e. Dilator
   f. Suture
2. 1% lidocaine
3. Povidone-iodine
4. Sterile gauze
5. Sterile gown, gloves, towels, sheets, hat, mask, and goggles
6. Sterile saline flush
7. Tegaderm or other clear occlusive dressing material
8. Blanket or towels to make a shoulder or neck roll
9. A nurse or technician to help

PROCEDURE

1. If you prefer, place a roll (towels folded up or a blanket rolled up) to make the vein more superficial. This roll is most useful for subclavian lines and is placed vertically between the scapulae. The bigger the person, the bigger the roll needed. Place the patient in the Trendelenburg position for the IJ or subclavian routes.
2. Clean the insertion site with povidone-iodine (or other agent). Begin scrubbing at the site of puncture and scrub outward to a diameter of 10 cm.
3. Next, put on your mask, hat, and goggles. Then wash your hands, put on your sterile gown and gloves, and drape the patient. Wait until the cleanser has air dried before draping. Remember that the drapes need to cover the entire patient. Just having the puncture area draped is inadequate.

4. Have someone hold the sterile flush for you. Draw it up into a syringe and flush all the ports of the line. Save some to flush the ports again once the line is in place.

5. Palpate the landmarks and then determine the location of your insertion point (see below for details). Infiltrate the skin with lidocaine using a small-gauge needle. Then advance the needle and infiltrate the subcutaneous tissues (and bone if subclavian route is chosen). Always draw back before injecting to make sure you are not inside a blood vessel.

6. Find the vein with the appropriate needle by advancing it slowly and continuously drawing back. Once you see blood in the syringe, go more slowly and continue to advance a few more millimeters until the flow is brisk.

7. Determine whether the blood is venous or arterial. If the patient is hemodynamically normal, venous blood is dark and under low pressure. In circumstances in which it is difficult to determine whether the blood is venous, several tests may be performed:

   a. Take the syringe off the needle and occlude the needle hub with your thumb. Briefly uncover the hub and watch for the color and pressure of blood that comes out. Do not leave the needle hub uncovered for more than a brief moment, as you may otherwise introduce air into the venous system, causing an embolism.

   b. Place a small catheter over the wire and into the vein to transduce the pressure. The waveform will tell you if it is arterial.

   c. Connect some sterile tubing filled with saline to the end of the needle and gauge the pressure by holding the tubing up in the air. Arterial blood will fill the tubing, whereas venous blood will not.

   d. Sending a blood gas will help in some situations. You can use the PO_2 (partial pressure of oxygen) to determine whether it is venous or arterial.

   e. Compare the blood you have withdrawn with some blood from the arterial line (if the patient has one).

   f. *Most important*, if you are unsure that it is venous, take out the needle and try again. Putting a large-bore catheter in the artery is always worse than trying multiple sites before cannulating the vein.

8. Place the wire through the needle into the vein. It is essential to **maintain control of the wire at all times.** Then remove the needle over the wire. (If a finder needle was used initially, first cannulate the vein with the larger needle and then place the wire.) Never force the wire. If it is within the vein, it will advance easily. You can dissect or perforate the vessel with the wire if excessive force is used. In addition, you should watch the heart rhythm as the wire is advanced. If it enters the heart, it can cause arrhythmias. If you see any ectopy, pull the wire back immediately.

9. Make a small puncture in the skin on top of the wire. This should be through the dermis only. Then slide the dilator over the wire. **Hold on to the wire.** The purpose of the dilator is only to make a subcutaneous tunnel through which the catheter can be placed. You therefore do not need to advance the dilator into the vessel, as doing so can cause the vessel to perforate. If you are placing a Cordis catheter, first place the dilator into the catheter and then advance both as a unit. Once in place, remove the dilator and wire together, leaving the catheter behind.

10. Take the catheter and advance it carefully over the wire. If you are using a triple-lumen catheter, remove the brown port cap, as the wire will exit through that distal port. Once you have a hold of the wire near the brown port, advance the catheter into the vessel. Depending on the person's body size and location of the puncture, you will need to advance the catheter a variable distance (generally 12–18 cm for IJ and subclavian, and all the way for femoral). The catheters are marked every centimeter. You want the tip to end up at the superior vena cava–right atrial junction for the IJ and subclavian routes.

11. Once the catheter is in place, remove the wire. Put the cap back on the brown port immediately to prevent air embolism. Test all ports for blood return, and flush each port. Then suture the catheter in place. Dress the site according to your institution's nursing policy.

12. For the subclavian and IJ routes, order a chest x-ray immediately.

13. Observe the site for bleeding and the patient for symptoms of shortness of breath, chest pain, or hypoxia that may indicate a procedural complication (e.g., pneumothorax, intrathoracic bleeding).

14. Look at the x-ray carefully. Look for a pneumothorax as well as for correct catheter placement. The tip of the catheter should be at the junction of the superior vena cava and the right atrium for IJ and subclavian lines. If the line is in too far, pull it back under sterile conditions and resuture it to the skin.

SITE-SPECIFIC PUNCTURES

Subclavian

To enter the subclavian vein, puncture the skin at a spot that is two-thirds of the way down the clavicle from the manubrium. This usually correlates to the place just medial to where the clavicle bends superiorly. Start 1–2 cm inferior to the clavicle. Your needle should enter the skin at this point. The angle of the needle should be such that the tip points toward the sternal notch. Find the clavicle with the tip of the needle, and then slowly walk your way down the bone until you are just under the bone. Then advance slowly while continuously drawing back. Keep the needle almost parallel to the skin surface.

Femoral

To find the femoral vein, first find the femoral arterial pulse; the vein will be just medial to this landmark. Enter the vein *below* the inguinal ligament. A good landmark is to go 2 cm inferior to the skin crease.

Internal Jugular

There are three different ways to enter the IJ. No matter what approach is used, always use a small (finder) needle to find the vessel before cannulating it with a larger-bore needle. In addition, have the patient's head turned away from the side of the puncture.

- Anterior approach (Fig. A4-1): This approach (A) enters the internal jugular vein at the medial edge of the sternocleidomastoid's medial head. At this level, the vein is just underneath the muscle belly and is very superficial. In a nonobese patient, your needle should only need to be advanced 2–3 cm. Place your free hand on the carotid pulse at the level of the cricoid ring. Then enter the skin just medial to the sternocleidomastoid and skive underneath the muscle. This will be approximately 5–6 cm above the clavicle. The angle of the needle should be pointing toward the ipsilateral nipple.

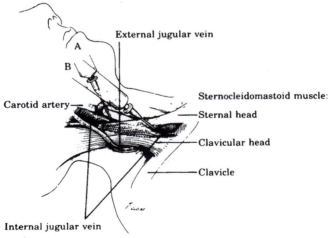

FIG. A4-1.
Internal jugular vein access approaches. **A:** Anterior approach. **B:** Central approach. (Reprinted with permission from Fries ES. Vascular cannulation. In: Kofke WA, Levy JH, eds. *Postoperative critical care procedures of the Massachusetts General Hospital.* Boston: Little, Brown, 1986.)

- Central approach (see Fig. A4-1): In this approach (B), you enter the vein closer to the clavicle. Your needle should enter the skin at the apex of the triangle formed by the lateral (clavicular) and medial (sternal) heads of the sternocleidomastoid muscle. Your needle should be aimed caudally and laterally toward the ipsilateral nipple.

- Posterior approach: The posterior approach is used rarely and has the highest risk of carotid puncture. The needle should enter the skin at the intersection of the lateral border of the clavicular head of the sternocleidomastoid and a line drawn laterally from the cricoid ring. Aim the needle caudally and anteriorly toward the sternal notch.

RULES FOR CENTRAL VENOUS ACCESS

1. Place central venous lines only when absolutely needed.
2. Attempt subclavian placement when there is no contraindication.
3. After three attempts at a single site, *stop* and call someone for help.
4. Always use sterile technique, draping patient and bed completely.
5. Always ensure that placement is *not* arterial before placing the dilator and catheter.
6. Maintain control of the wire at *all* times.
7. For the subclavian and IJ routes, check a chest x-ray immediately and adjust line position as needed. Always obtain an x-ray, even if the placement attempt was unsuccessful. If unsuccessful, do not attempt the contralateral side without first ruling out a pneumothorax by x-ray.

5 Paracentesis

Nirmal K. Veeramachaneni

The usual indication to perform paracentesis is in both the diagnostic and therapeutic management of ascites. Before inserting a needle into a patient's abdomen, recognize the contraindications and pitfalls:

1. Prior abdominal surgery may lead to adhesions and bowel scarred to the abdominal wall. Avoid going through a prior surgical incision. When in doubt, perform this procedure under ultrasound imaging guidance.
2. One cause of ascites is hepatic failure, with concomitant coagulopathy. The patient may require transfusion of platelets or FFP before this procedure to prevent bleeding. Check for coagulopathy before the procedure.

SUPPLIES

Prepackaged kits are available. Otherwise, the materials required include

1. Sterile gauze sponges
2. Sterile gloves and drapes
3. Povidone-iodine or other skin cleansing agent
4. 1% lidocaine
5. Long angiocath (16 or 18 gauge for therapeutic aspiration, or a smaller gauge for diagnostic, small-volume aspiration)
6. Sterile tubing with a three-way stopcock
7. Vacuum bottles or sterile tubes (depending on the amount of fluid to be removed)

PROCEDURE

1. Have the patient void beforehand or place a Foley catheter.
2. Look for abdominal incisions and percuss the abdomen for fluid level (area of dullness).
3. The usual location for paracentesis is in the midline or in the lateral position. Midline insertion should be midway between the umbilicus and symphysis pubis, with attention to avoid areas of tympany (bowel floats). Lower quadrant insertion is typically done in a triangle bounded by the lateral border of the rectus sheath, a line from the umbilicus to the anterior superior iliac spine, and the anterior superior iliac spine to the symphysis pubis.

4. Clean the insertion site with povidone-iodine (or other agent). Begin to scrub at the site of paracentesis and scrub outward to a diameter of 10 cm.

5. After the cleanser has air dried, place the sterile drapes.

6. Infiltrate the skin and subcutaneous tissue with lidocaine. Always draw back before injecting to make sure you are not inside a blood vessel.

7. Insert the Angiocath through the skin only, and then change the angle by shifting the needle in a different direction before entering the peritoneal cavity. Doing so creates a nonlinear needle track and helps prevent leakage of ascites after the procedure. Using constant negative pressure, advance the needle. You will feel resistance when the fascia is encountered.

8. As soon as ascites is encountered, *stop* advancing the needle. Advance the plastic angiocath, aiming for the pelvis.

9. Attach either a sterile syringe for diagnostic fluid sampling or tubing fitted with a three-way stopcock. This tubing may then be connected to a vacuum bottle.

10. Use caution when aspirating large volumes. Removal of large-volume ascites may require IV volume resuscitation with crystalloid or albumin. Slowly remove large volumes over an hour.

11. At the conclusion of the procedure, remove the catheter and apply a dry, sterile dressing. A purse-string stitch may be required at the skin site for persistent leakage of ascites.

6 Thoracentesis

Nirmal K. Veeramachaneni

Like paracentesis, thoracentesis may be performed for therapeutic as well as diagnostic purposes. Similar to paracentesis, relative contraindications include coagulopathy, small effusions, prior surgery, or organized infection. Beware of the pulmonary cripple—patients with such poor pulmonary reserve that they will not tolerate a pneumothorax. Additionally, a chest CT or ultrasound imaging may be required in those with complicated effusions.

SUPPLIES

Prepackaged kits are available. Otherwise, the materials required include

1. Sterile gauze sponges
2. Sterile gloves and drapes
3. Povidone-iodine or other skin cleansing agent
4. 1% lidocaine
5. Syringes and needle (22 gauge for diagnostic, 18-gauge Angiocath for therapeutic)
6. Sterile tubing
7. Vacuum bottles or sterile tubes (depending on the amount of fluid to be removed)

PROCEDURE

1. In preparing to do the procedure, review the x-ray, and have the film at the bedside. Examine the patient carefully. Identify the transition from tympany to dullness on percussion.
2. In the awake, cooperative patient, have him or her lean over a table or tray, with the back exposed (Fig. A6-1A).
3. The intubated patient should be properly sedated with the security of the endotracheal tube ensured and then placed in the lateral decubitus position with the effusion in the dependent position. Repeat the exam, and confirm the location of dullness.
4. Clean the insertion site with povidone-iodine (or other agent). Begin to scrub at the site of thoracentesis and scrub outward to a diameter of 10 cm.
5. After the cleanser has air dried, place the sterile drapes.

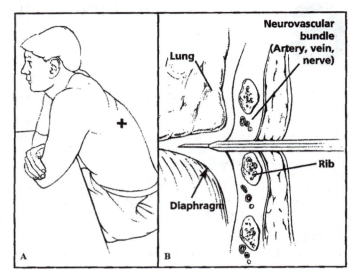

FIG. A6-1.
Thoracentesis. **A:** Positioning in the conscious patient. **B:** Needle is advanced over the rib to avoid damaging the neurovascular bundle.

6. Infiltrate the skin and subcutaneous tissue with lidocaine. Always draw back before injecting to make sure you are not inside a blood vessel.

7. Thoracentesis should be done in the posterior axillary line, below the level of the effusion. Take care when performing this procedure below the ninth rib, as it is possible to enter the abdominal cavity. The needle puncture should be above the rib to avoid injury to the neurovascular bundle found on the inferior aspect of each rib (Fig. A6-1B).

8. Slowly insert the needle. Maintain constant negative pressure. It helps to have a small quantity of lidocaine in the syringe to anesthetize the periosteum as you "walk" over the rib with the needle.

9. Once inside the pleural space (confirmed by the aspiration of pleural fluid), stop advancing the needle. In the case of a therapeutic tap, advance the plastic angiocatheter over the needle. Aim for a dependent position and remove the needle. Many of the commercially available kits contain a one-way valve that is activated once the needle is removed from the catheter. Otherwise, be careful not to allow air to enter the pleural space. Various collection containers may then be attached to the catheter; often, sterile tubing connecting the catheter to a large syringe or to a sterile vacuum container is used to facilitate drainage.

10. In the event of air being aspirated during the initial attempt, withdraw the needle. This event signifies entry into the lung. Repeat the thoracentesis in a more dependent position.
11. When adequate fluid has been removed, remove the needle or catheter quickly, maintaining constant negative pressure.
12. Apply a sterile dressing.
13. All patients should have a chest x-ray to rule out pneumothorax or hemothorax.
14. Reexpansion-induced pulmonary edema may result from removal of large quantities of fluid, so be cautious in removing >1 L of fluid at a time.

7

Chest Tube

Nirmal K. Veeramachaneni

The chest tube is a common drainage procedure in the treatment of pneumothorax, effusion, hemothorax, or chylothorax. The specific type of tube used depends on the indication. Like all procedures, placement of a chest tube is not without risk. Complications include injury to lung, injury to vessels, and improper positioning, such as into a pulmonary fissure. When done electively, it is important to check first for underlying coagulopathy. Often, however, chest tubes are placed emergently.

SUPPLIES

Prepackaged kits are often available. When they are not, the minimum requirements are
1. Sterile gauze sponges
2. Sterile gloves and drapes
3. Povidone-iodine or other skin cleansing agent
4. Syringe and needle
5. 1% lidocaine
6. Scalpel
7. Two large Kelly clamps
8. Appropriate sized chest tube
   a. Pneumothorax (24–32 French)
   b. Hemothorax, chylothorax (32–40 French)
9. Needle driver and 2-0 or 3-0 silk suture
10. Petroleum-impregnated gauze
11. Adhesive tape
12. Suction
13. Device to provide water seal, regulate suction, and collect fluid
    a. Traditional 3-bottle system
    b. All-inclusive containers, such as Pleurovac

PROCEDURE

1. Patient positioning is essential. The patient should be supine or lateral and as close to the edge of the bed as possible for adequate exposure. Place a towel roll under the scapula if the patient is supine. The arm should be abducted above the head. The usual location to insert a tube is in the fifth rib space, in the anterior axillary line. The male nipple or lower third of the scapula serves as a guide. This position avoids excessive patient discomfort and

allows the patient to rest in a supine position without compressing the tube. Also, the risk of placing the tube in the abdomen or into the liver is reduced.

2. Clean the insertion site with povidone-iodine (or other agent). Begin to scrub at the site of incision and scrub outward to a diameter of 10 cm.

3. After the cleanser has air dried, place the sterile drapes.

4. Infiltrate the skin and subcutaneous tissue with lidocaine. Always draw back before injecting to make sure you are not inside a blood vessel.

5. Like with thoracentesis, the chest tube will be placed above the rib to avoid injury to the neurovascular bundle. Anesthetize the periosteum of the rib, as well as the pleural space. You may do so by entering the pleural space with the needle under constant negative pressure. When you encounter air or pleural fluid, slowly pull back. When you are no longer able to aspirate air or fluid, administer the anesthetic agent into the parietal pleura.

6. A 1- to 2-cm incision is made at the inferior aspect of the rib below the entry rib space. Many recommend blunt dissection into the rib space above the incision. This is done to create a tunnel and help prevent air leak. An alternate method is to provide skin/subcutaneous tissue traction superiorly with the nondominant hand and incise directly to the level of the rib (this technique avoids a great deal of painful blunt dissection, allows direct visualization, and still provides a degree of tunneling of the chest tube, helping to prevent air leak).

7. A Kelly clamp is then directed above the rib, into the pleural space (Fig. A7-1A). A gush of fluid or air is often evident.

8. Open the clamp to create a large enough hole to allow entry of your index finger. Insert your finger to confirm entry into the pleural space and to sweep away any adhesions that may be present (Fig. A7-1B).

9. Clamp the distal (nonfenestrated) end of the chest tube to avoid drainage of pleural contents on insertion.

10. Guide the proximal (fenestrated) end into the chest using the second clamp (Fig. A7-1C). Proper placement usually means superiorly and posterior. This allows adequate drainage of fluid when the patient is supine. Anterior placement may be done for evacuation of a pure pneumothorax.

11. Connect the chest tube to the source of suction/water seal.

12. The tube must be secured to the patient. A silk purse-string suture helps ensure a tight seal around the tube. An additional stitch from the corner should be placed to further secure the tube. Secure the tube according to your institution's technique, as it will help avoid confusion if someone else removes it.

13. Apply the petroleum-impregnated dressing and gauze to the insertion site. Apply tape to the connection points in the tubing to prevent accidental disconnection. Be liberal with the tape (Fig. A7-1D).

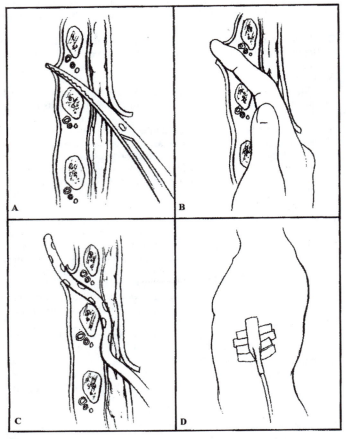

FIG. A7-1.
Chest tube insertion. **A:** A Kelly clamp is inserted over the rib into the pleural cavity. **B:** The index finger confirms the tract and sweeps away pleural adhesions. **C:** Chest tube path. **D:** Secure taping of the chest tube.

14. Perform a chest x-ray to confirm proper placement. The last side hole in the tube interrupts the radiopaque line found on chest tubes. Make sure this last hole is completely inside the pleural cavity on x-ray.

15. Pain management is essential after a chest tube is placed, as it is one of the most uncomfortable bedside procedures.

8 Endotracheal Intubation

Jeremy Goodman

An endotracheal tube may be placed in the unconscious, nonbreathing patient in the course of CPR or in any patient demonstrating worsening respiratory status and requiring mechanical ventilation.

SUPPLIES

1. Endotracheal tube
   a. 8.0–9.0 mm cuffed for the average male
   b. 7.0–8.0 mm cuffed for the average female
2. Stylet
3. Laryngoscope handle with blade
   a. Macintosh blade is curved.
   b. Miller blade is straight.
   c. Number 3 or 4 size for average adults.
4. 10-mL syringe
5. Suction equipment with Yankauer attachment
6. Water-soluble lubricant
7. Magill forceps
8. Tape
9. Bag-valve mask
10. End-tidal CO_2 device (if available)
11. Oral or nasal airway

PROCEDURE

1. If time and patient condition permit, preoxygenate the patient with 100% oxygen by bag-valve mask for several minutes before intubation. The unconscious patient should have an oral or nasal airway placed.
2. Check all equipment:
   a. Extend laryngoscope blade and confirm that light works.
   b. Inflate endotracheal tube cuff with 10 mL air to check for leak and then deflate.
   c. Lubricate the distal end of the tube.
   d. Lubricate the stylet and place it through the lumen of the endotracheal tube, and mold into a gentle curve. Make sure the stylet does not extend past the distal end of the tube.
   e. Confirm proper function of suction equipment.

3. Place the patient in the "sniffing position" (neck flexed, head extended) unless contraindicated owing to cervical spine injury.
4. Have an assistant hold cricoid pressure.
5. Hold the laryngoscope in your left hand and open the patient's mouth with your right hand.
6. Remove the oral airway, if present.
7. Insert the laryngoscope blade into the right side of the mouth and advance, while gently sweeping the tongue to the left.
8. Use suction to clear secretions and the Magill forceps to clear foreign bodies.
9. Advance the laryngoscope blade to the epiglottis.
10. The tip of the curved blade is placed anterior to the epiglottis in the vallecula (Fig. A8-1A). The tip of the straight blade is placed below the epiglottis (Fig. A8-1B).
11. When lifting the laryngoscope handle, do not lever back against the teeth. Instead, lift straight up and forward.
12. Once the vocal cords are visualized (Fig. A8-2), gently pass the endotracheal tube through them until the cuff is just beyond them.
13. *Do not spend >30 secs trying to place the endotracheal tube.* Once 30 secs have elapsed, remove the laryngoscope and reventilate the patient with the bag-valve mask before attempting to intubate again.
14. Remove the stylet and attach the bag-valve mask.
15. Inflate the cuff with 5–10 mL of air. Once the cuff is inflated, cricoid pressure may be released.
16. An end-tidal CO_2 device may be interposed between the tube and the bag-valve mask to confirm placement in the airway.
17. Auscultate over both lung fields and the stomach to confirm proper placement of the tube in the airway. Diminished or absent breath sounds over the left chest suggest that the tube is advanced too far and lies in the right main bronchus. Deflate the cuff, withdraw the tube 1–2 cm, and reinflate the cuff. Auscultate for breath sounds again.
18. Tape the tube in position.
19. Confirm tube placement with a portable chest x-ray.

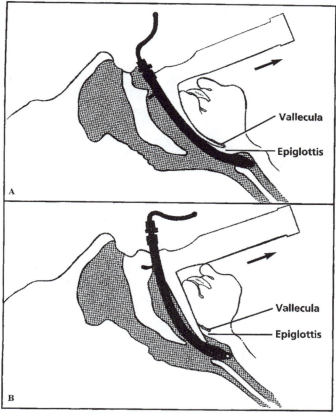

FIG. A8-1.
Laryngoscope positioning for endotracheal intubation. **A:** The curved-blade tip is placed in the vallecula. **B:** The straight-blade tip lifts the epiglottis from a posterior direction.

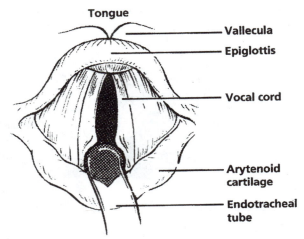

FIG. A8-2.
View of the vocal cords as seen on direct laryngoscopy.

Common Templates

B

Jeremy Goodman

PREOPERATIVE NOTE

- Name of procedure
- Indication for procedure
- Preoperative testing results (CBC, chemistry, coagulation studies, urinalysis, chest x-ray, ECG)
- Status of blood bank products (type and screen or cross)
- Diet status (NPO after midnight)
- Consent status (signed and in chart)

DICTATED OPERATIVE NOTE

- Preoperative diagnosis
- Postoperative diagnosis
- Surgeon
- Assistants
- Operative procedure performed
- Anesthetic technique
- Preoperative indications for procedure
- Description of procedure
  - Positioning of patient
  - Incision
  - Findings
  - Technique
  - Type of closure
- Complications
- Sponge and needle count
- Fluid management (inputs and outputs) and blood products transfused

- Estimated blood loss
- Patient disposition and condition at end of procedure (including pertinent details, e.g., peripheral pulse exam after vascular surgery)

BRIEF OPERATIVE NOTE (FOR CHART)

- Preoperative diagnosis
- Postoperative diagnosis
- Surgeon
- Assistants
- Anesthetic technique
- Brief description of relative findings
- Complications
- Drains placed
- Fluid management
- Estimated blood loss
- Patient disposition and condition

POSTOPERATIVE NOTE/DAILY NOTE

- Name of procedure (and postoperative day)
- Subjective
  - What the patient tells you
- Objective
  - Vital signs
  - Ins and outs
  - Physical exam
- Lab and microbiology data
- Medications, including days since start of each antibiotic
- Assessment
- Plan

ADMISSION ORDERS

- Admit to
  - Location, attending name, service
- Diagnosis

- Condition
  - Stable, guarded, critical
  - Code status
- Vitals
  - Frequency of vital sign measurements
- Activity
  - Ad lib, bed rest with bathroom privileges, bed rest with bedside commode, bed rest, head or extremity elevation, weight-bearing status
- Allergies
- Nursing
  - Strict inputs and outputs, tube care, drain care, dressing changes
- Diet
- IV fluids
- Medications
  - Antibiotics
  - Pain medications
  - Ulcer prophylaxis
  - Deep venous thrombosis prophylaxis
  - Home medications
  - PRN medications
- Labs
- Studies
  - Radiology, vascular lab, cardiac lab
- Other
  - Physical/occupational/speech therapy, dietitian, social worker

DISCHARGE NOTE

- Attending surgeon
- Date of admission
- Date of discharge
- Diagnoses
- Procedures performed

APPENDIX B: COMMON TEMPLATES

- History on admission
- Physical exam on admission
- Lab and radiology studies on admission
- Hospital course
- Discharge instructions
  - Medications
  - Follow-up
  - Activity
  - Diet
- Status on discharge

ACLS Algorithms

All figures are reprinted with permission from Lippincott Williams & Wilkins. Web address is: http://circ.ahajournals.org/cgi/content/full/102/suppl_1/I-136 [*Circulation* 2002;102(supplement I):I-136–I-165].

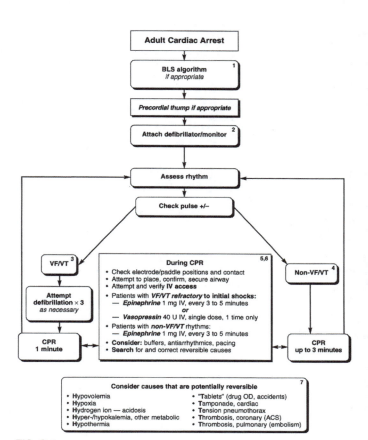

FIG. C-1.
ILCOR Universal/International ACLS algorithm.

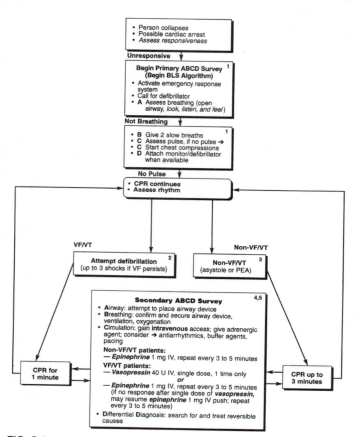

FIG. C-2.
Comprehensive ECC algorithm.

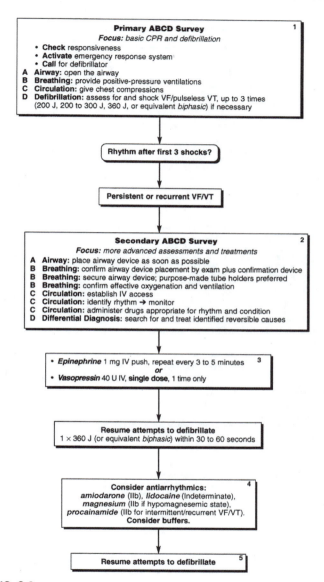

Primary ABCD Survey 1

Focus: basic CPR and defibrillation

- **Check** responsiveness
- **Activate** emergency response system
- **Call** for defibrillator

A **Airway:** open the airway
B **Breathing:** provide positive-pressure ventilations
C **Circulation:** give chest compressions
D **Defibrillation:** assess for and shock VF/pulseless VT, up to 3 times (200 J, 200 to 300 J, 360 J, or equivalent *biphasic*) if necessary

Rhythm after first 3 shocks?

Persistent or recurrent VF/VT

Secondary ABCD Survey 2

Focus: more advanced assessments and treatments

A **Airway:** place airway device as soon as possible
B **Breathing:** confirm airway device placement by exam plus confirmation device
B **Breathing:** secure airway device; purpose-made tube holders preferred
B **Breathing:** confirm effective oxygenation and ventilation
C **Circulation:** establish IV access
C **Circulation:** identify rhythm → monitor
C **Circulation:** administer drugs appropriate for rhythm and condition
D **Differential Diagnosis:** search for and treat identified reversible causes

- *Epinephrine* 1 mg IV push, repeat every 3 to 5 minutes 3
  or
- *Vasopressin* 40 U IV, **single dose, 1 time only**

Resume attempts to defibrillate
1 × 360 J (or equivalent *biphasic*) within 30 to 60 seconds

Consider antiarrhythmics: 4
amiodarone (IIb), *lidocaine* (Indeterminate),
magnesium (IIb if hypomagnesemic state),
procainamide (IIb for intermittent/recurrent VF/VT).
Consider buffers.

Resume attempts to defibrillate 5

FIG. C-3.
Ventricular fibrillation/pulseless ventricular tachycardia algorithm.

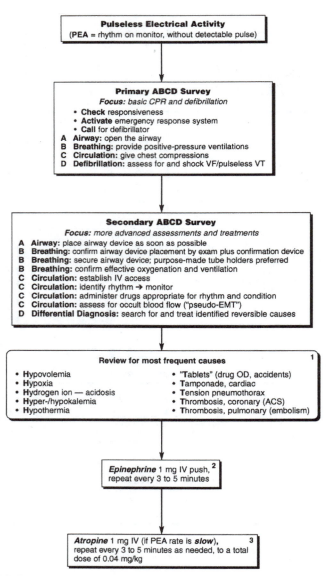

FIG. C-4.
Pulseless electrical activity algorithm.

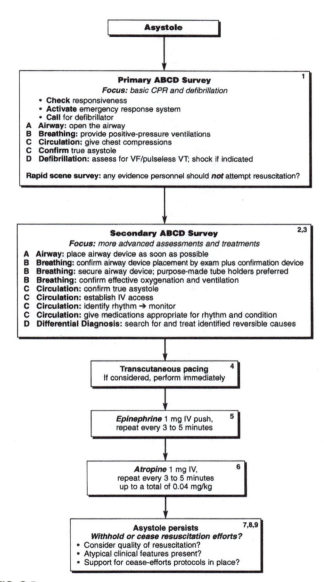

FIG. C-5.
Asystole: the silent heart algorithm.

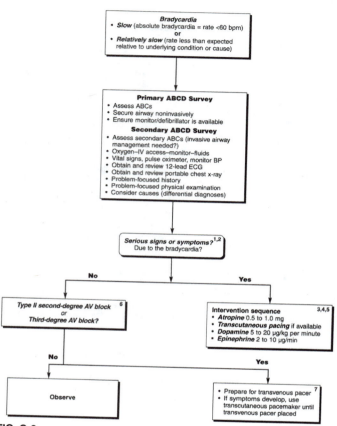

FIG. C-6.
Bradycardia algorithm.

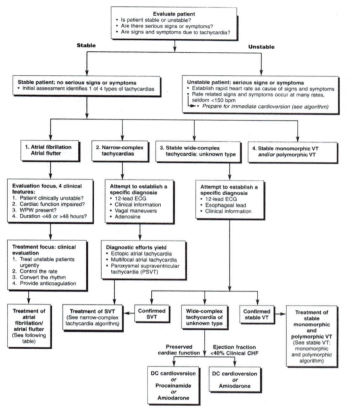

FIG. C-7A.
The tachycardia overview algorithm.

Control of Rate and Rhythm (Continued From Tachycardia Overview)

Atrial fibrillation/ atrial flutter with • Normal heart • Impaired heart • WPW	1. Control Rate		2. Convert Rhythm	
	Heart Function Preserved	Impaired Heart EF <40% or CHF	Duration <48 Hours	Duration >48 Hours or Unknown
Normal cardiac function	Note: *If AF >48 hours' duration, use agents to convert rhythm with extreme caution in patients not receiving adequate anticoagulation because of possible embolic complications.* *Use only 1 of the following agents (see note below):* • Calcium channel blockers (Class I) • β-Blockers (Class I) • For additional drugs that are Class IIb recommendations, see Guidelines or ACLS text	*(Does not apply)*	**Consider** • DC cardioversion *Use only 1 of the following agents (see note below):* • Amiodarone (Class IIa) • Ibutilide (Class IIa) • Flecainide (Class IIa) • Propafenone (Class IIa) • Procainamide (Class IIa) • For additional drugs that are Class IIb recommendations, see Guidelines or ACLS text	• **NO DC cardioversion!** • **Note:** *Conversion of AF to NSR with drugs or shock may cause embolization of atrial thrombi unless patient has adequate anticoagulation.* • Use antiarrhythmic agents with extreme caution if AF >48 hours' duration (see note above). **or** **Delayed cardioversion** Anticoagulation × 3 weeks at proper levels • Cardioversion, then • Anticoagulation × 4 weeks more **or** **Early cardioversion** • Begin IV heparin at once • TEE to exclude atrial clot **then** • Cardioversion within 24 hours **then** • Anticoagulation × 4 more weeks
Impaired heart (EF <40% or CHF)	*(Does not apply)*	Note: *If AF >48 hours' duration, use agents to convert rhythm with extreme caution in patients not receiving adequate anticoagulation because of possible embolic complications.* *Use only 1 of the following agents (see note below):* • Digoxin (Class IIb) • Diltiazem (Class IIb) • Amiodarone (Class IIb)	**Consider** • DC cardioversion **or** • Amiodarone (Class IIb)	• **Anticoagulation** as described above, followed by • **DC cardioversion**
WPW	Note: *If AF >48 hours' duration, use agents to convert rhythm with extreme caution in patients not receiving adequate anticoagulation because of possible embolic complications.* • DC cardioversion **or** • **Primary antiarrhythmic agents** *Use only 1 of the following agents (see note below):* • Amiodarone (Class IIb) • Flecainide (Class IIb) • Procainamide (Class IIb) • Propafenone (Class IIb) • Sotalol (Class IIb) **Class III** **(can be harmful)** • Adenosine • β-Blockers • Calcium blockers • Digoxin	Note: *If AF >48 hours' duration, use agents to convert rhythm with extreme caution in patients not receiving adequate anticoagulation because of possible embolic complications.* • DC cardioversion **or** • Amiodarone (Class IIb)	• DC cardioversion **or** • **Primary antiarrhythmic agents** *Use only 1 of the following agents (see note below**):* • Amiodarone (Class IIb) • Flecainide (Class IIb) • Procainamide (Class IIb) • Propafenone (Class IIb) • Sotalol (Class IIb) **Class III** **(can be harmful)** • Adenosine • β-Blockers • Calcium blockers • Digoxin	• **Anticoagulation** as described above, followed by • **DC cardioversion**

WPW indicates Wolff-Parkinson-White syndrome; AF, atrial fibrillation; NSR, normal sinus rhythm; TEE, transesophageal echocardiogram; and EF, ejection fraction.

Note: Occasionally 2 of the named antiarrhythmic agents may be used, but use of these agents in combination may have proarrhythmic potential. The classes listed represent the Class of Recommendation rather than the Vaughn-Williams classification of antiarrhythmics.

FIG. C-7B.
Control of rate and rhythm (continued from tachycardia overview).

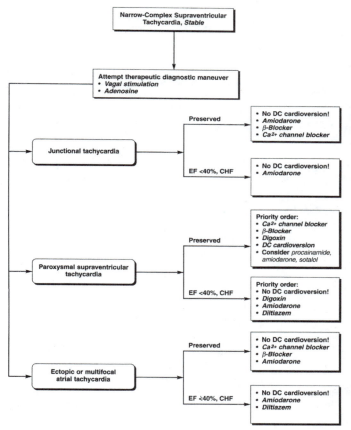

FIG. C-8.
Narrow-complex supraventricular tachycardia algorithm.

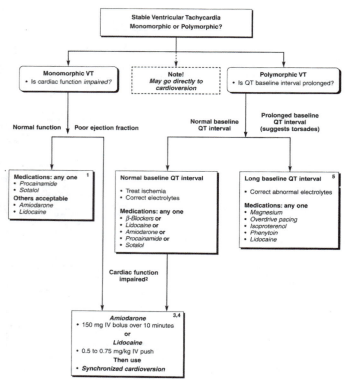

FIG. C-9.
Stable ventricular tachycardia (monomorphic or polymorphic) algorithm.

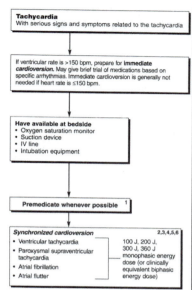

Tachycardia
With serious signs and symptoms related to the tachycardia

If ventricular rate is >150 bpm, prepare for **immediate cardioversion**. May give brief trial of medications based on specific arrhythmias. Immediate cardioversion is generally not needed if heart rate is ≤150 bpm.

Have available at bedside
- Oxygen saturation monitor
- Suction device
- IV line
- Intubation equipment

Premediate whenever possible   1

Synchronized cardioversion   2,3,4,5,6
- Ventricular tachycardia
- Paroxysmal supraventricular tachycardia
- Atrial fibrillation
- Atrial flutter

100 J, 200 J, 300 J, 360 J monophasic energy dose (or clinically equivalent biphasic energy dose)

Notes:
1. Effective regimens have included a sedative (eg, *diazepam, midazolam, barbiturates, etomidate, ketamine, methohexital*) with or without an analgesic agent (eg, *fentanyl, morphine, meperidine*). Many experts recommend anesthesia if service is readily available.
2. Both monophasic and biphasic waveforms are acceptable if documented as clinically equivalent to reports of monophasic shock success.
3. Note possible need to resynchronize after each cardioversion.
4. If delays in synchronization occur and clinical condition is critical, go immediately to unsynchronized shocks.
5. Treat polymorphic ventricular tachycardia (irregular form and rate) like ventricular fibrillation: see ventricular fibrillation/pulseless ventricular tachycardia algorithm.
6. Paroxysmal supraventricular tachycardia and atrial flutter often respond to lower energy levels (start with 50 J).

Steps for Synchronized Cardioversion
1. Consider sedation.
2. Turn on defibrillator (monophasic or biphasic).
3. Attach monitor leads to the patient ("white to right, red to ribs, what's left over to the left shoulder") and ensure proper display of the patient's rhythm.
4. Engage the synchronization mode by pressing the "sync" control button.
5. Look for markers on R waves indicating sync mode.
6. If necessary, adjust monitor gain until sync markers occur with each R wave.
7. Select appropriate energy level.
8. Position conductor pads on patient (or apply gel to paddles).
9. Position paddle on patient (sternum-apex).
10. Announce to team members: *"Charging defibrillator—stand clear!"*
11. Press "charge" button on apex paddle (right hand).
12. When the defibrillator is charged, begin the final clearing chant. State firmly in a forceful voice the following chant before each shock:
    - *"I am going to shock on three. One, I'm clear."* (Check to make sure you are clear of contact with the patient, the stretcher, and the equipment.)
    - *"Two, you are clear."* (Make a visual check to ensure that no one continues to touch the patient or stretcher. In particular, do not forget about the person providing ventilations. That person's hands should not be touching the ventilatory adjuncts, including the tracheal tube!)
    - *"Three, everybody's clear."* (Check yourself one more time before pressing the "shock" buttons.)
13. Apply 25 lb pressure on both paddles.
14. Press the "discharge" buttons simultaneously.
15. Check the monitor. If tachycardia persists, increase the joules according to the electrical cardioversion algorithm.
16. Reset the sync mode after each synchronized cardioversion because most defibrillators default back to unsynchronized mode. This default allows an immediate defibrillation if the cardioversion produces VF.

FIG. C-10.
Synchronized cardioversion algorithm.

Patient Data
Tracking Form

Name	
DOB	Age
Admission date	Attending

<u>HPI</u>

<u>PMH</u>   <u>PSH</u>

<u>Home meds</u>   <u>Allergies</u>

Admission vitals/labs

T	HR	BP	RR
SaO$_2$		Ht	Wt
Ca	Bili$_T$	Alk Phos	PT
Mg	AST	Amylase	INR
Phos	ALT	Lipase	PTT

Other labs

UA

ECG

CXR

CT

Other Rads

<u>Procedures/Events</u>   <u>Dates</u>

Last name:

Date	POD	Date	POD
Overnight Events		Overnight Events	
T_{max}	SaO_2	T_{max}	SaO_2
HR	BP	HR	BP
Invasive hemodynamics		Invasive hemodynamics	
Vent settings		Vent settings	
Ins		Ins	
Outs		Outs	
IV fluid type/rate		IV fluid type/rate	
Lines (day)		Lines (day)	
Drains (day)		Drains (day)	
Antibiotics (day)		Antibiotics (day)	
Diet		Diet	
Other labs		Other labs	
Studies		Studies	
Plan		Plan	

Index

Page numbers followed by *f* indicate figures; page numbers followed by *t* indicate tables.